The Best of Times

Also by Nicole Meredith

Outsights: Inequality from Inside and Out (with Lorne Tepperman)

Waiting to Happen: The Sociology of Unexpected Injuries
(with Lorne Tepperman)

The Best of Times

Nicole Meredith

Rock's Mills Press
Oakville, Ontario
2020

Published by
Rock's Mills Press
www.rocksmillspress.com

For information about this book, contact us at:
customer.service@rocksmillspress.com

Contents

A Pandemic-Era Preface

When is the best time to have a baby? That is one of the questions this book tries to answer, using recent demographic and sociological research. Figuring out the answer was never simple to begin with, but it was made much more complicated by the COVID-19 pandemic, which burst upon the world as *The Best of Times* was partway through production.

Initially, as physical distancing, work-from-home advisories, and lockdowns kept couples cooped up at home together, some joked that a baby boom was on the horizon. At the same time, many health care professionals advised couples to temporarily postpone starting a family if possible, as the effects of the virus on pregnant women and babies were relatively unknown.

Amidst all this uncertainty, one thing did seem certain: the health care system was overburdened. Even urgent medical appointments, including some cancer treatments and essential surgeries, were postponed to free up health care workers and hospital beds for COVID-19 patients, and this pattern has repeated itself wherever subsequent waves of the pandemic have flared up. As this preface is being written, the number of COVID-19 cases in Canada and many other countries has dropped dramatically, foreshadowing some form of return to a "new normal," if not the old pre-pandemic normal. But unless and until either a reliable vaccine or effective treatment for the novel coronavirus is rolled out on a wide scale, new outbreaks seem inevitable. What does all of that mean for people who are thinking about having a baby? As the pandemic continues to unfold, will pregnant women be able to get prenatal care, ultrasounds, and other medical attention when and where they need them? What will our hospitals look like? Will they be able to provide optimal care for mothers and their newborns? And what will be the consequences for hopeful would-be parents of some fertility clinics postponing new treatment cycles, as occurred in the early stages of the pandemic?

But couples planning to have children aren't just grappling with medical questions. The widespread economic disruption caused by the pandemic left many Millennials facing a second "once-in-a-lifetime" financial crisis in barely a decade, the Great Recession of 2008–09 being, of course, the first. Their already shaky finances crumbled. Some who may have been toying with the idea of starting a family no longer felt financially ready. Others found themselves living with mom and dad once again, having been laid off and unable to pay rent. Starting or maintaining the kind of serious relationship that might lead to having a baby can prove difficult if you lack independence, privacy, and financial stability. And others say they'd rather stay single until things calm down; virtual or physically-distanced dates don't appeal.

None of these patterns are new. COVID-19 has exacerbated them and drawn greater attention to them, but for many years now, Millennials have been feeling the pressures of a precarious labour market, moving back home to live with their parents and staying single into their thirties. That's why, despite the significant and still-evolving implications of COVID-19, it is important to emphasize that both the research that forms the foundation of this book, and the conclusions that research supports, remain valid. Before the coronavirus appeared, I argue, there was a "best" time to have your first baby, and that remains the case during the pandemic—as it will once the pandemic subsides. No doubt adjustments in plans and timing depending on individual economic and medical circumstances will need to be made, and as you read through the pages that follow, you will undoubtedly come across passages that harken back to a time before anyone had ever heard of the term "social distancing." But in the end, even in what have all too often seemed the worst of times, there still is a "best of times" to have a baby—and that is what this book is all about.

NICOLE MEREDITH
August 2020

The Best of Times

INTRODUCTION
Later Baby

The Mindy Project was an American TV sitcom about a group of OB/GYNs, featuring quirky, successful Princeton graduate Mindy Lahiri (played by actor and comedian Mindy Kaling). In the show's third season, she takes a hiatus from her New York-based practice to accept a fellowship at Stanford, where a friend shows her an empty office space and asks: "How would you feel about starting a world-class fertility clinic here?" Mindy spends the remainder of the episode fighting with her boyfriend, Danny, about whether they should move across the country before she learns she's (very unexpectedly) pregnant. Chaos erupts as she takes dozens of pregnancy tests, avoids telling Danny, gets outed by his mother at an awkward family dinner, moves into his apartment, debates having what he calls a "quickie shame wedding," and doesn't even dream of telling her parents she's "knocked up," all while ironically opening her own fertility clinic where she'll help other couples conceive.

In an effort to acquire more patients, Mindy begins a program called "Later Baby" which, in her words, is meant "to convince girls in their twenties to want to freeze their eggs." She travels around to university campuses pitching the service to female students, to whom she explains: "When I was your age, I thought that I was going to be married by the time I was twenty-five. But it took a lot longer than that. And unfortunately, your body does not care if you are dating the wrong guy... Your body, and your eggs, just keep getting older. Which is why freezing them is actually a pretty smart idea, because it gives you a little more time so you can try to find that one diamond in the crap heap of American men." Her presentations receive thunderous applause, and Later Baby's success is ultimately the reason Mindy's able to keep her clinic afloat—even after she has her own son.

Many viewers found *The Mindy Project* endearing because it put a light-hearted twist on issues they genuinely cared about. Are "egg freezing" and artificial insemination the way of the future, now that so many young women stay in school well beyond their twenties? (After all, when she discovered she was pregnant, Mindy was a stably employed thirty-something in a long-term relationship with an equally successful fellow doctor. Would the decision to keep her baby have been so easily made if she had just started medical school? Or if she were still in high school?) What should you do if you find yourself unexpectedly pregnant? And most importantly: When *is* the best time to have a baby?

My purpose in writing this book is to answer that question, using recent demographic and sociological research. Before I go any further, though, I need to clarify what I'm promising to tell you in the coming pages. More accurately, I need to explain what I'm *not* going to do. I'm not going to tell *you*, specifically, when to have your first baby. I'm not going to do that for several reasons:

1.   Plenty of people are already trying to tell women how to live their lives and what to do with their bodies, as we'll see in the upcoming chapter about birth control. I think women are perfectly capable of making their own decisions. So, I don't want to be among those prescriptive people.

2.   Even if I tried to tell you when to have your first baby, I wouldn't get it right. In the pages that follow, you'll see just how many factors combine to shape women's fertility decisions—everything from your upbringing and relationship with your parents, to your race and income, to your political views and personal values. Some of these variables drive women to have children at ages or life stages that, according to the research we'll look at, are suboptimal. Think of teenagers who have babies because they were raised to believe abortion is wrong. Or women who grew up with abusive parents, so they marry and have children later than average to feel sure about their choice of a partner. Or those who know their job prospects and income will never improve, so they reason there's no point putting off a family until they earn more. In short, every woman

brings unique life experiences that make the best time to have a baby a little different for everyone. That means I can't tell *you* when to have your first kid, because I don't know you, your life, or your goals.

3. I'm not presumptuous enough to think you'd make this life-changing decision based on what you read in this book. You probably already have your mind made up—or at least, you probably already have a general sense of what you'd like your future to look like. This book isn't necessarily intended to change that plan.

Instead, this book is meant to help you think about having children in some fresh new ways. I look at the most popular ages and life stages for having babies, and ask *why* women decide to have kids when they do. I also consider what women want—as opposed to what they end up doing—and ask if they would opt to have kids at a different point in their lives, given the option. And I ask: what age and life stage carries the best chances that both mother and child will lead the healthiest, happiest lives?

First Babies and a Model

The decision to have a child is actually a series of decisions. We can make sense of these decisions by organizing them chronologically and making use of a simple framework that we'll call the *WiSK model*. "WiSK" is an acronym, where W = wants a child, S = starts a child, and K = keeps a child. What we want to figure out is how and why women come to want, start, and keep a child at different points in their lives.

For convenience, let's call the different life stages in which these decisions are made and acted upon *Early* (ages 15 to 24), *Middle* (ages 25 to 34), and *Late* (ages 35 to 44). In the coming chapters, I compare the attitudes and decisions of women from these different age categories.

For example, of women aged 16, 28, and 40, how many want a first child? How many intend to get pregnant in the near future—say, within the next three years? How many actually *do* get pregnant in that time? How many abandon their initial decision if they don't get pregnant? Among those who conceive, how many keep the child, abort it, or give it up for adoption?

Unsurprisingly, we will see that far more women want, start, and keep babies in the Middle and Late stages than in the Early stage. But we'll also see less "typical" patterns and ask: what leads women of different ages to want but not start babies? Or to want and conceive but not keep babies at these different ages? Why do some women change their minds about wanting to have a child, and why do others never want children at all? And what are the differences between women who intentionally get pregnant and those like Mindy, who just don't *prevent* getting pregnant?

As mentioned, the answers to these questions lie in a complicated interaction of social factors. These include a woman's level of education, career plans, job status, relationship status, housing situation, and so on. The answers also have to do with larger-scale things like the availability of affordable, high-quality childcare, and paid parental leave.

These decisions will also be influenced—although less consciously—by social norms and expectations about parenthood. Whether we recognize them or not, "standards" exist about what age and life stage it's "appropriate" for people to have children. Some are widely accepted: for example, few people believe 15-year-olds should be having children. Others are muddier: for example, should people only have kids if they're married? After they're finished school? Once they own a house? I devote an entire chapter to exploring these social pressures, where I ask whether women *believe* they are expected to have kids by a certain age, or after they have accomplished certain life goals, and if those expectations are strong enough to make them have children by those benchmarks.

I also consider whether some women make WiSK decisions because of a lack of such expectations. Young women who grow up in neighbourhoods where teen pregnancy is common, post-secondary education is rare, and unemployment is high aren't constrained by the same norms as those whose parents expect them to build successful careers *before* having kids. So, not all women in the Early group avoid starting a child, or abort accidentally conceived ones; the timing and sequencing of WiSK events differs among women of different races, socioeconomic backgrounds, from urban versus rural areas, and who grew up living with different family members in different household arrangements.

After exploring all of these scenarios and variables, we will see that different childbearing decisions lead to different outcomes. For example, women who have their first child in the Early, Middle, and Late years tend to have different parenting styles and concerns. Age at first birth can also predict the total number of children a woman has—in other words, how large her family is in the end. In turn, these parenting styles and family sizes can impact the health and happiness of parents and children alike. So, the important conclusions we'll reach at the end of this book have to do with answers to the questions:

1.   How are children affected by the relative age of their mother?

2.   Are mothers from one of these age groups more likely to be healthier and happier?

3.   Are mothers who were finished school, stably employed, and married when they had their first child more likely to have these good outcomes for themselves and their kids?

By answering such questions, I want to empower women—including you, the reader, if you are confronting these choices—with the information needed to feel confident about their WiSK decisions. So many Millennials' ears are ringing with the voices of their parents, grandparents, in-laws, co-workers, friends, and countless others who all seem to be wondering if and when they'll "finally" start a family. If you've ever been on the receiving end of the "When I Was Your Age…" monologue or the "When Are You Going To Give Me A Grandchild?" interrogation, I hope this book will give you some fresh perspectives and statistics to fire back with. I also hope it will help you feel less alone, by showing you that plenty of women—and men—are facing the same fears, weighing the same pros and cons, and making many of the same choices.

CHAPTER ONE

Deviation and Delays: New Norms in the Millennial Life Course

At age 26, Julia Barrett finally moved out of her mother's house. She had been living at home while in school, but after graduating, Julia couldn't find a job that would pay her rent: "If I moved out at that point … I would be in an apartment with no money." It wasn't until two years later that Julia had the financial stability she needed to fly the coop.[1]

The remarkable thing about Julia's story is that it is unremarkable. Today, it's the new normal: roughly four in ten people age 20–29 live with their parents.[2] Like Julia, they can't find a job, or they're saddled with massive student debts that make paying the rent feel impossible. Living with mom and dad seems like the reasonable—even responsible—thing to do.

But a few decades ago, Julia would have been an outlier. "Growing up" has changed a lot in recent years. People take longer to reach milestones, like moving out, that were traditionally seen as markers of adulthood. One of these milestones is having a baby: it's taking women longer today to take this big step than ever before. As it turns out, starting a family while living in your parents' basement isn't a popular choice.

This chapter is all about growing up in the twenty-first century. I look at what people expected from life a generation ago: when they expected to move out, marry, and have children, and the order they expected those things to happen in. Then, I look at how young adults today think about these life choices: when—or if—they expect to move out, settle down with a partner, and start a family. As with every generation, there's a divide here. Baby Boomers and Millennials head down different paths through life, arguing all the while about whose route is better. This chapter weighs the pros and cons of each path, to help people decide which is right for them.

Questions you'll get answers to:

▶ *Why are Millennials taking new paths through life—that is, different paths than their parents probably took?*

▶ *Is one path through life better than another?*

▶ *How are these changing paths affecting fertility?*

Some Sociological Groundwork

Sociologists call paths through life "life courses." As years go by, people pass through different stages: childhood, adolescence, adulthood, old age.[3] Each stage brings different experiences and responsibilities:[4]

- Childhood is a time for being innocent and carefree.
- Adolescence is when you go to school and start "finding yourself."
- Adulthood means getting a job, marrying, and having children.
- Old age brings retirement, leisure time, and grandchildren.

The version of life captured in these bullet points is pretty whitewashed and western. In, say, Namibia, the life course would look different. And if we were in the seventeenth century, it would look different too. In every society and time period, people transition physiologically from childhood to adolescence to adulthood. But the things they expect—and the things expected of them—during each of those phases change.[5] That's because our social, cultural, and economic surroundings change. For example, when the economy shrinks and jobs become scarce, people finishing school struggle to transition from "student" to "employed adult" as quickly. As we adjust to these changes, we also adjust our expectations of what we should be doing at different ages and phases in the life course.

The Many Metaphors of Life

As the western life course evolves, so do the metaphors sociologists use to describe it. Some of my personal favourites:

- For Baby Boomers, life is a highway. And middle age is rush hour on that highway: the career you're trying to build, the kids you've got to raise, and the aging parents you're supposed to take care of are all slowing you down, all at once.
- For Millennials, life is more like the Parisian public transit system: sprawling, confusing, and always under construction.
- You can always venture off the beaten path, but it won't be as easy as cruising down the highway.

Here's how sociologists unpack each of these metaphors:

In the 1960s, '70s, and '80s, people took the highway version of life: a straightforward, predictable route that was similar for everyone.[6] People would finish high school, go on to college or university, get a stable job, marry, and start a family.[7] In those days, good jobs were widely available, housing was more affordable, and marriage and children were the norm.[8]

Today, we have the public transit system version of life. A variety of routes take people to many different destinations.[9] Some people stay in school until they're in their thirties. Others put off school and go backpacking through Europe instead. Others, like Julia, may *want* a life like their parents', but find it takes longer to secure a career and a home of their own.

In the last few decades, growing up has changed so much that sociologists have created an entirely new phase in the life course: emerging adulthood. Julia is a prime example. When she finished school at age 23, she was technically an adult, if we consider her age alone. But she had yet to make several key transitions: she still lived with her mom, couldn't support herself financially, and didn't know what kind of career she wanted. Julia was thus in a transitional phase: old enough to be considered an adult, but still struggling to behave the way we expect "adults" to.

In typical sociological fashion, we had to come up with another metaphor to describe this new development. In keeping with the transportation theme, emerging adulthood has been deemed a bridge. It connects the total dependency of childhood with the independence of adulthood. Decisions made on this bridge are crucial: they determine what the rest of life looks like. Most people today find themselves on the bridge when they're between 18 and 30. And during this phase, they find themselves experiencing many big role changes one right after another. They go from being dependent children, to semi-independent students, to part-time wage earners, to full-time career pursuers, to dating partners, spouses, and first-time parents. But after all of that madness happens in a few short years, people inhabit the same roles for decades. Unless you get divorced and/or remarried, the next big role change will typically come 30 or 40 years later, when most people retire. So, to repeat, decisions made on the bridge are decisions that shape the rest of our lives.

Baby Boomers and Millennials

The bridge phase of life is also forcing people to recognize generational differences. That is because, as Julia can attest, it extends the time that people of different generations live under the same roof. Decades ago, most people would have moved out of their parents' homes by age twenty. But today, many parents have front row seats to their grown children's struggle: they know exactly what these emerging adults are doing, because they live in the same house. Most are supportive, but others are perplexed or frustrated, chiding their children to finally "grow up".[10] In some cases, close living quarters spark intergenerational conflicts, laying bare the different ways older and emerging adults view life.

Let's classify these older adults—the parents of today's emerging adults—as Baby Boomers. (Bear in mind the start and end dates of generations are flexible and loosely defined). Born post-World War II, these Baby Boomer parents are in their fifties or sixties now. They grew up expecting to travel the highway version of life because that's what *their* parents experienced. And, for the most part, they've followed precisely that life course. Once they finished school, most were able to find jobs, buy houses, marry, and start a family because they were coming of age at a time of economic prosperity.[11]

Baby Boomers were also raised to see the world—and their place in it—a certain way. This outlook impacted every piece of the WiSK process. First, Baby Boomer women (and men) *wanted* kids because they had been taught that women's main responsibilities were as homemakers and mothers. Bigger families were also more popular back then: most couples *wanted* at least two or three children. So, they would typically start trying to have kids in our Early phase, or in the younger years of our Middle phase. Very few had a reason *not* to start trying; they weren't busy finishing school or starting a career. Finally, Baby Boomers were living in an age of post-war prosperity. They could afford to *keep* unwanted pregnancies, even if they'd already had the two or three children they'd originally planned for. In sum, Baby Boomer women wanted, started, and kept babies at high rates, leading to larger families overall.[12]

On the highway of life, Baby Boomers should be enjoying retirement by now (or at least getting ready for it). But some are coming up against a roadblock: they can't retire because their own children haven't moved out yet.

These emerging adults are part of the Millennial generation (also known as Generation Y). Born between the mid-'80s and 2000s, Millennials are in their twenties and thirties today. Many, like Julia, have never left their parents' homes at all. Others have been dubbed "Boomerang kids": they move into dormitories while in school, only to return to their parents' homes after graduating.

Essentially, Baby Boomers and Millennials expect different things from life. Some Baby Boomers can't understand why their children aren't scrambling to settle down and start a family. Some Millennials complain their parents won't stop nagging them about all the things they had done by the time they were in their twenties or thirties. Parents and children often butt heads on what's "normal" because, to repeat, the "right" life course is always changing. And it has changed substantially in Millennials' lifetime.

The Right Age or the Right Life Stage

Millennials weren't the original travellers of the winding path through life. Plenty of others have had their highway version of life interrupted. These interruptions often reveal how people feel about ages and life stages. The men who returned home from World War II, bringing the Baby Boom with them, are a perfect example.

Instead of working towards milestones like graduation and finding their first job, these men had been on the battlefield. After the war was over, many of them had to go back to school, even though they were older than the average student. As a result, statistics from that time period show that men finished school and start working at older ages, compared to the men of the previous generation.[13] Yet, the average age at which they got married stayed the same. In other words, these men weren't putting marriage off until they finished school, and thereby sticking to the usual *order* of the life course. Instead, they were getting married at the *age* they were expected to.

For Baby Boomers (and many generations before them), life events were tied to particular ages. You were supposed to be finished school by a certain age, married by a certain age, and starting a family by a certain age. People still thought there was a correct order in which to do these things. But, as the data shows, people who grew up in the post-war years would often do them in the "wrong" order so they could do them by the "right" age.

Today, the opposite rule seems to apply: Millennials are trying to do things in the right order, instead of by the right age. They stay in school and live with their parents longer, making them like the post-war generation who had to start and finish school later. But unlike those post-war adults, Millennials don't mind putting off marriage (or kids). In the 1950s and '60s, the median age for a first marriage was 20.3 years for women, and 22.8 years for men. In 2004, the median age was 25.1 years for women and 26.8 years for men. So, the desired ordering of events across the life course has stayed the same; it's the length of time people are taking on average to accomplish those events that's changing.[14]

Of course, some Millennials are doing things in the "wrong" order, mostly because it's taking them longer to hit milestones.[15] With so many pursuing master's and doctoral degrees, some Millennials marry before they're finished school. Others insist on finding their dream job before settling down with a life partner, only to find themselves in their late thirties, single, and worried their biological clock is running out. They may become single parents, skipping the marriage milestone altogether.

For the most part, though, even Millennials want the conventionally ordered life course.[16] Doing things in the "wrong" order can have negative consequences.[17] Mostly, that's because we have social structures to support life course transitions at the "normal" ages, in the "normal" order.

Take the transition from high school to university as an example. Universities try to make that transition easier in many ways. For one, they hold first-year seminars that resemble the small classes of high school. They also offer on-site dormitories where students can get help from each other and from dons, as they try living away from their parents for the first time. And frosh week is designed to be fun for 18-to-20-year-olds. Mature students don't benefit as much from these support systems, because the systems weren't designed with them in mind.

So, when people diverge from the expected path through life, there are fewer supports to help them. And without those supports, they are at a greater risk of failing.[18] For example, people who marry before finishing school or starting their careers are more likely to wind up in unstable relationships, and eventually break up.[19] People who put off post-secondary education after high school finish less school overall, and accordingly earn less, even when their socioeconomic backgrounds are taken into account.

Becoming pregnant at the "wrong" time can also have negative consequences.[20] The words "teen mom" inspire dread almost universally. Adolescent girls who keep their babies are less likely to finish high school, let alone go to college or university. That greatly reduces their chances of having a rewarding career, and being financially stable. In fact, having a baby as a teenager increases a woman's chances of ending up on welfare, and people who marry in an attempt to legitimate their unplanned pregnancy are more likely to divorce.

In short, people enjoy support when they follow a "normal" life course, and they often endure negative consequences when they deviate from it. That's enough to make most people conform: to follow the path through life that we're raised to believe is "normal."

Learning the Life Course

From the time we're born, we're subtly taught to think there's a proper order in which to do things in life, and a proper age at which to do them. We learn this unconsciously, by hearing about and observing our parents' lives, and by watching our siblings grow up. We also see our friends act differently when they reach certain ages (and we witness the consequences). And as I'll spend an entire chapter of this book discussing, we take note of what's portrayed as normal, weird, funny, or terrifying in movies and on TV.[21]

The "normal" life course is the easy one to follow. It's the highway version of life: the paved road that's just waiting for us to take it. It's easy to travel, and that makes it appealing to most. But if you decide to drive off the highway, you're going to have to deal with potholes, steep drop-offs, and trees blocking your way. Essentially, you'll come up against barriers if you try to forge your own path through life. These barriers include judgment by others, ridicule, disapproval, and even exclusion.[22]

Even if you've never been the target of shaming, you know what would inspire it. Getting pregnant in high school is a prime example. Girls know their parents would be furious, and they'd lose at least some friends. They want to avoid the negative social consequences that come with taking that less-travelled path. So, for the most part, they avoid getting pregnant.

In this sense, our path through life is more predetermined than we like to imagine. It's instilled in us while we grow up, and structured by what we fear others will think about us.[23] The highway is thus the textbook version of what life is "supposed" to look like. It's what many think is "normal," and it's how many behave as they grow up.

But, as the transit system metaphor implies, more Millennials *have* been choosing their own paths.[24] They take detours, like backpacking through Europe before taking their first job. Others go backwards, moving back in with their parents after university. Others still have created new pathways altogether, founding start-ups instead of taking a nine-to-five job. That means we're at an interesting point in history: a turning point in life course development. Lots of emerging adults are venturing off the beaten path. But their parents are only starting to get used to the idea.[25]

Soon, Millennials' seemingly eccentric, "immature" behaviour will become the new norm. Throughout history, young people have sparked changes to the dominant life course. Such changes begin when people start accepting unconventional behaviours, while still behaving conventionally themselves. Gradually, larger numbers of people become willing to behave in those formerly unconventional ways. By the time the formerly unconventional behaviours become customary, even proponents of convention have accepted them.

We're already starting to see this happen. True, many Baby Boomers still say that Millennials take too long to grow up. But others wonder if they're merely being responsible: maybe it *is* best to finish school and get a job before moving out. Few parents today would say that Millennials should cut their education short so they can marry at a "normal" age. So, Millennials are coming of age when our understanding of the life course is in flux. Some expect them to conform to the traditional trajectory that Baby Boomers know and love. But others are starting to accept a delayed transition to adulthood—especially if it means more education and a better job in the long run.

The Cohabitation "Crisis"

Just a few decades ago, pre-marital cohabitation was widely unacceptable.[26] If you wanted to move in with your boyfriend or girlfriend, chances are your parents would freak. This was—and still is—especially the case in religious, conservative families. These families may even see cohabitation as a sin: an acknowledgment that you're having sex before marriage.

Fast forward to today, and cohabitation is the new norm. A majority—roughly 70 percent—of married couples live together before tying the knot.[27] As cohabitation becomes increasingly popular, three things are happening more and more often: some people are having babies later, some are having babies outside of marriage, and some aren't having babies at all.[28]

First, some people are having babies later because cohabitation often delays milestones. Many treat it like a "trial" marriage. They see moving in together as a stepping stone in their relationship: a way to test their commitment and see if it's what they really want. This new desire to test has a lot to do with rising divorce rates. Many Millennials watched their parents struggle through divorces; they want to avoid that suffering for themselves, and ensure they've found the right partner before marrying them.[29]

Research shows this is a wise approach. It's becoming increasingly unlikely that your first cohabitation will lead to marriage. And the length of time spent in that first cohabitation has shortened, on average.[30] In other words, it's becoming less and less likely that you'll marry the first partner you live with. It's also taking people less time to figure out they don't want to marry that person. Good thing they tested the waters before taking the plunge.

But thanks to this trial period, many couples are having babies later. Decades ago, people would only move out of their parents' house when they were getting married.[31] And as we've seen, they were pretty young—in their early twenties—when that happened. But today, it's completely normal for youth to try other living arrangements.[32] They may boomerang back into their parents' houses, find their own apartment, or live with roommates. *Then*, they may devote several more years to living with a partner before marrying. Moving through these different living arrangements takes time, thereby pushing back the point at which young adults feel ready to start thinking about children. (These experimental living situations can take up so much time, some scholars think we should count them as yet another new phase of the life course.[33] They just haven't come up with a catchy metaphor for it, yet.)

The second thing that's becoming more common is having kids outside of marriage. Until roughly the 1950s, almost everyone who had a child was married. Most people married first and had a baby second; and women who got pregnant accidentally would often marry their partners to legitimate the pregnancy. But today, a growing number of parents just cohabit.[34] And some studies show that cohabiting couples are *more* likely to have a baby outside of wedlock.[35]

Some—including the aforementioned religious and conservative people—would say this is a crisis. They think our culture's new endorsement of cohabitation is actually an endorsement of pre-marital sex. And they point to births among unmarried cohabiters as evidence that couples should wait until they are married before moving in together. In reality, those couples may have made a conscious choice to have children without marrying.[36]

Regardless, the data show that there is certainly not a cohabitation crisis. The majority of people say they would prefer to marry before having children.[37] And most births in Canada today are to married couples.[38] So, the rising prevalence of cohabitation is not destroying the institution of marriage, nor is it popularizing common-law parenthood.

Third and finally, some cohabiters are less likely than married couples to have children. There are two main "types" of people in this group. The first are generally liberal, secular people with less traditional values. They don't value marriage, so they don't marry. And their less traditional values and lifestyles also translate into a desire to stay child-free. Sometimes these are couples who choose to make their work or their relationship or other important things in their lives the priority.

The second group are couples who don't plan to stay together in the long term. Maybe they just live together because it's cheaper to split the bills. Or maybe one partner is staying with the other while she finds a place of her own. The way these couples stumble into cohabitation—rather than actively making plans for their future together—creates inertia. They may rely on each other financially and emotionally; and because they share housing and expenses, it's harder for them to break up. But because they are only committed to each other for practical reasons, they report being dissatisfied with their relationships. They are unlikely to make the long-term commitment of having a child together—at least, not on purpose.

In sum, cohabitation is much more common today than it was in the past. But it hasn't replaced marriage. The majority see cohabitation as a temporary arrangement. Within five years of moving in together, 90 percent of cohabitations have ended: the couples have either broken up or married.[39] Nor has cohabitation substantially changed people's preference for being married before having children.

What Does This Mean for Fertility?

If the life course is now more like public transit than a highway, then where does childbearing fit in? The main thing we have seen in this chapter so far is that it's taking people longer and longer to reach "adulthood." And until people reach certain milestones associated with adulthood, they are less likely to think about starting families of their own, let alone make the other decisions in our WiSK model.

Across the developed world, the average age at which women have their first child has been steadily climbing since the late 1960s. In the early 1970s, the average age was 24 or 25; now it is 28 or 29 in OECD countries.[40] In Canada, mothers are having their first birth, on average, when they are over 30 years old.[41] Moreover, women are having fewer children overall, in their lifetimes.[42] Today, fertility rates in OECD countries are below replacement level.[43] That means people aren't having enough children to replace themselves, and the population will decline overall. The fertility rate is climbing slightly today, but as you can see in the chart below, fertility in the early 2000s was at its lowest point in much of Europe since World War II.[44]

In sum, women are having fewer babies today. They are also having their first child at older ages.[45] Why? There are two main reasons: higher education and work opportunities.

First, more people are getting a post-secondary education than ever before.[46] That education demands lots of time and attention, for at least several years.[47] For that reason, most women postpone marriage—let alone having kids—until they've finished school.[48]

Figure 1
Fertility Rates in Selected Countries, 1950–2020

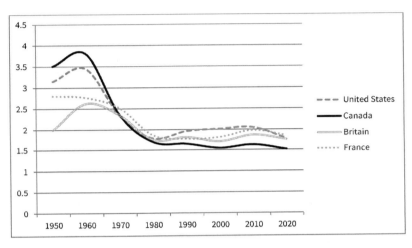

Source: Data compiled from macrotrends.net.

Figure 2
Women's Age at Birth of First Child, Western Europe and United States, 1980–2005

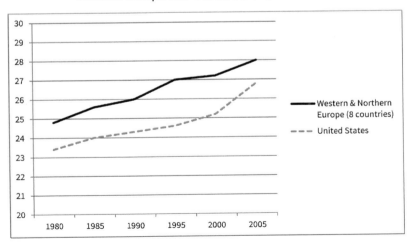

Source: Based on Frejka and Sobotka (2008), *Demographic Research* 19 (3): 15–45.

That's why, on average, more highly-educated women have their first children at older ages.[49] Likely, the number of women who postpone childbearing will continue to grow, as the number of jobs that require post-secondary education rises.[50]

It's worth noting that men often follow a similar thought process. Most want to land a stable job that would support their partner and children. One study found that married men enrolled in school were 25 percent less likely to have a first child than married men not enrolled in school.[51] So, men typically postpone childbearing until they've graduated and started working.[52]

As well, higher education can broaden people's horizons. It might instill new values, desires, and ambitions.[53] At least some forms of higher education teach students to value their own personal fulfillment over social conformity. In other words, it may help students think critically about what's expected of them. And it might encourage them to pursue paths in life other than the socially sanctioned highway version of life.

So, education can help women see that they have more options available to them in life than becoming a wife and mother. Women whose worldviews are changed by education may pursue other goals first, before having children. Or they may decide they don't want children at all.[54] As education makes women eligible for rewarding, high-paying work, they may become less willing to take time away from that work to have a child. More on this to come.

Finally, higher education can reduce two common barriers to divorce: stigma and financial dependence. Higher education can soften people's views on divorce, making them more willing to leave their relationship if it becomes unsatisfying.[55] Higher education also gives many women the means to support themselves financially. So, they don't *need* to stay in an unsatisfying marriage because they lack alternatives. This is largely a good thing: women (and men) shouldn't feel trapped in unhealthy relationships. However, it can force highly-educated women to postpone their childbearing plans indefinitely: they might divorce right when they would have otherwise started a family. By then, it may be too late for them to find a new partner, re-marry, and begin the WiSK process before their biological clock runs out.

The second factor pushing back the average age at which young people start having children is the rise of women at work.[56] In every country, fertility rates decline as female labour force participation rises.[57] In 1960, the female labour force participation rate in OECD countries was 41 percent, and the average total fertility rate was 2.9. By the late 1990s, the female labour force participation rate had climbed to 64 percent, while the average total fertility rate had dropped to 1.6.

At first glance, these statistics seem to confirm a big fear people had in the 1950s. Back then, people thought that women who worked would inevitably have fewer children. After all, it's hard to balance a career and kids. So, as more women began working fulltime, even researchers assumed they would postpone childbearing, have fewer children overall, or avoid having children altogether.[58]

This logic seems to hold today, according to the statistics above: when female employment rates go up, fertility rates go down. Surprisingly, though, researchers have shown that's not actually what's happening.[59] Consider the data on childbearing across different countries. We could reasonably expect fertility rates to be lowest where female employment is highest—yet the *opposite* is true.[60] In countries like New Zealand, the U.S., Norway, and many Western and Northern European countries, there are high rates of female participation in the labour force. Yet, in those same countries, fertility rates have now returned to around replacement levels.[61] By contrast, in Southern European countries like Italy and Spain, many young women are unemployed or stuck in low-paying, unstable jobs. There, the fertility rate remains low.[62] Why?

The answer has to do with the *type* of work women can get. On the one hand, women can raise overall household income by working, making it easier to financially support a child. But on the other, having a child carries an "opportunity cost".[63] That is, you risk missing out on opportunities and gains at work by having a child instead.

Working women know that, to have children, they'll need

to interrupt their work at some point. They also know that interruption will reduce their long-term earnings in at least one of three ways.[64] First, they'll lose income during the time they take off to give birth and care for their newborn. The exact amount of lost income will depend on how much paid maternity leave the new mother is eligible to receive, but even the best benefits packages pay new mothers far less than their original salary. Second, during that maternity leave, the new mother is missing out on promotion opportunities. That loss that will reduce the rate at which her salary grows in the future. Third, a woman's prolonged absence from work may cause her skills, knowledge, and experience to decline. While legislation bans employers from firing pregnant women or mothers on maternity leave, those who return to work unable to perform may be dismissed. The risk is especially big if new mothers prove unable to fulfill their responsibilities at work because of new demands their child is placing on their time and energy.

Women take all three of these consequences into account when making WiSK decisions. Their current wages, their predicted future wages, and the wages they risk losing after having a baby all shape women's perception of the viability of starting a family. Women in relationships also do similar cost-benefit analyses of their partner's job stability and income. Some conclude their husband's salary alone would be enough to support a family.[65] In those cases, women who work for the pay, rather than because they want a rewarding career, may care less about these opportunity costs. On the other hand, choices are more constrained when a couple's combined incomes are barely enough to raise children with.

These low incomes are characteristic of part-time, unstable, temporary positions. Think cashiers, bartenders, and retail workers, for example. Many people accept this work when they can't get anything better, as when jobs are scarce and unemployment is high. In these circumstances, people are more likely to (accurately) expect losing income as a result of having a baby. They know their bartending job won't be waiting for them in a few months. And if there were only a few of these jobs to begin with, the chances of getting a new one are slim.

This uncertainty makes planning a child risky and unappealing to most precarious workers.

So, when unemployment rates are high and people are afraid to briefly leave the labour market, fertility rates decline. This has been shown to be true for men and women alike. If both partners are trapped in precarious jobs, chances are they don't feel confident about their ability to afford a baby.

By contrast, in communities with low unemployment rates, fertility rates are at or close to the replacement level.[66] This is especially the case when there is plenty of social support, and the labour market easily accommodates exits and re-entries.[67] Where jobs are strongly protected for people who leave and return to the labour market, and where maternity leave packages are generous, the costs of having a baby are lower. In these contexts, women know their jobs will be waiting for them when they return from maternity leave, and that they will be getting some compensation during that period of leave.

For these reasons, fertility rates are lower in countries with high rates of unemployment and precarious work. Fertility rates dip especially low when women are concentrated among the unemployed and precariously employed.[68] In these circumstances, women put off childbearing so they can:

- acquire more skills,
- reduce their risk of becoming "unemployable" while they're on maternity leave, and
- increase the level of income they can expect to enjoy for the rest of their lives.

Some realize they may have to abandon their desires for children altogether to keep even these unstable jobs.

There is one main exception to this rule. Some women become unemployed, but recognize they will likely be able to find a good job again in the future. In these cases, women may take the opportunity to have a child while they can, before seeking that next job. Even still, the promise of future employment is more common in societies with low unemployment rates and plenty of good opportunities. So, contrary to 1950s expectations, stable employment for women may *promote* childbearing—not stunt it. In an economy where most couples need to be dual earning to make ends meet, both men and women need good jobs to feel confident they can support a family. Women who can't find work, or who fear losing the precarious work they do have, seem to be the ones who don't actualize their dreams of having kids.

The Paradoxes of Progress

Changes to the life course take some getting used to. As we adjust to the new realities of prolonged higher education and women at work, some paradoxes have emerged. For example, highly educated women with good jobs have more to lose if they take time off work to have kids. Yet, childbearing rates are often high among highly educated women. As explained above, stably employed women are more likely than precariously employed or unemployed women to have babies.[69] The catch is, highly-educated, stably employed women have their kids at older ages.

This isn't only because highly-educated women are waiting to finish school before starting a family. It also has to do with the maternity leave benefits available to them. If a fixed allowance is allotted, the sheer existence of this allowance encourages working women to have babies. When they are younger or new to the work force, their wages are the lowest they will ever be. That means the fixed amount will make the greatest difference in boosting their overall earnings. Other women receive benefits in the form of a replacement rate over previous wages. In this case, the higher their earnings, the higher the benefits they'll receive. Because workers typically enjoy higher earnings the longer they work—gaining experience, skills, promotions, and raises over time—women who expect to receive replacement rates have an incentive to delay having a child. Working now gives them a chance to get promotions and raises, which means higher benefits when they have a baby later down the line.

To repeat, these considerations are fairly new: they're emerging because our highway version of life is morphing into the public transit system version of life. In the past, most women were financially dependent on men. They relied on their fathers to provide for them as they grew up and then they relied on their husbands once they were old enough to marry.[70] To ensure their financial stability, women had to solidify their marriages through childbearing. They would exchange unpaid labour (i.e., childcare and housekeeping) for financial support from their husbands. But since the mid-twentieth century, women have had alternatives. Access to higher education and paid work have meant women no longer *have* to entrust their livelihood to their husbands, and in turn, no longer *have* to bear children.

No wonder then, that some researchers find fertility rates and female oppression are related.[71] They suggest that, in unequal societies, women are denied work opportunities so they can prioritize housekeeping and childrearing. In these circumstances, fertility rates should rise. According to this theory, fertility rates naturally fall in Western egalitarian societies, where women and men (theoretically) enjoy equal educational and occupational opportunities. But they are naturally high in societies where women are expected to be wives and mothers, and nothing else.

As we have seen, this isn't the whole story. In a genuinely equal society, men and women would share household and child care responsibilities evenly. In that world, a woman who wants to pursue an education or a demanding career could still have as many children as she wants. But this is not how our world works. Women in western societies do not share the burdens of childbearing or child care equally with their partners. In turn, higher education and employment still affect women's childbearing decisions.

If men and women spent equal amounts of time caring for their children, they would be equally free to choose how much education they would get, the career they would pursue, and the timing at which they would start a family. Shared childcare responsibilities would allow women to balance their various roles—as working professional, wife, and mother—just as men have always done, instead of forcing them to choose between their careers and families. So, we do not live in a completely equal society. That means we cannot mistake reduced fertility rates as evidence of greater gender equality. Rather, they reflect an ongoing form of gender *inequality*: namely, an insistence that women are ideal homemakers and caregivers. If they are going to get an education and work, we seem to believe that women should not do so at the expense of the other roles they have filled in the past.

These high expectations we have for women are known as "having it all": enjoying the rewards of marriage, motherhood, *and* a successful career. With a few key adjustments to the life course, I believe that women really can have it all. Those key adjustments are the main topic of interest in the pages to come.

Final Thoughts

Low, below-replacement-level fertility rates have important implications for everyone—not just cash-strapped Millennials who can't afford to have as many children as they may like. To function properly, societies need to have balanced proportions of young, middle-aged, and old people. But if every couple has fewer than two children over the next several decades, our overall population will start to age more quickly.[72] The proportion of older adults in our society will outstrip the proportion of young and middle-aged adults.

In such age-imbalanced societies, young and middle-aged adults are put under a great deal of financial pressure. This is because health care, social security, and pensions are costly.[73] And the more people who need these social supports, the greater the burden on tax-paying adults to provide them. As a result, funds that might otherwise support parents and their children are devoted instead to health care and pensions for older adults.[74] For example, cash benefits for families may be cut, or the duration of paid parental leave may be shortened. And without these benefits, young adults may be even more reluctant to start families. A vicious cycle emerges, whereby too few babies causes an aging population, which causes a re-allocation of social funding that leads to even fewer babies.

In short, we have a so-called "demographic time bomb" on our hands: an aging population that could put unsustainable pressure on our health and social programs.[75] To dismantle that time bomb, we need to better understand the factors that shape people's fertility decisions, so we can support replacement level fertility rates.

As we have seen in this chapter, those factors are many and varied. The moment when a couple decides to have a baby is not an isolated incident. That decision is just one moment in a series of intertwined experiences we call the life course. Recognizing the many twists and turns in each individual life course helps put into perspective the many variables that play into the decision to have a child.

After all, it's one of the most important decisions people make in their entire lives. Part of the reason Baby Boomers equate parenthood with "growing up" is that it's irreversible.[76] People can "take back" other changes we typically associate with adulthood. As we've seen in this chapter, they can move back in with their parents after living on their own, or go back to school after trying a "real job." But women can't reverse having their first child, even if they decide not to keep it.

In other words, the choice to have a child is unique because it's unrepeatable. Anyone can marry a second (or third) time, or buy another home, but becoming a parent is a one-time life event. So, having a child signals a permanent, irreversible transition into parenthood. In North America, parenthood defines people's identities for most of their lives. Once you become a parent, you change your name to "Mom" or "Dad," and you keep that title until you die. Finally, parenthood demands a substantial investment of a mother's time, energy, money, and other resources. So, it will permanently limit the roles and opportunities open to her (and to her partner).

To determine why women have children when they do, we need to look at how they lived their lives before they even started thinking about becoming mothers.[77] The length of time women spend *not* being mothers—and the ways they occupy that time—can predict the type of mother they'll become. Not mothering can allow women to finish their education, establish their careers, pursue their dreams of travelling, find the right partner, buy a house, and segue into the more mature, adult phase of the life course.

In this sense, the older ages at which many women are having their first child may be beneficial all around. Older, more mature, and more highly educated women may be better able to provide high quality care and support for their children. They may also be able to negotiate more equal care arrangements with their partners, and balance their family responsibilities with their work ones.

We know the Baby Boomer generation believed in the highway version of the life course. We also know their Millennial children are not following that life course as often. They don't view it as necessary or desirable, and feel free to take the variety of routes sociologists have described as a sprawling public transit system. Lastly, we know Millennials' divergence from the formerly "normal" life course has led them to start their own families later in life. In turn, the average age at which Millennials become parents is older than that of the Baby Boomer generation.

What we *don't* know is how this changing life course will affect Millennials' future happiness and life satisfaction, and the well-being of their children. Because they are taking extra time to "grow up," mature, figure out what career path they truly want to pursue, and begin building some savings, Millennials may be stable and secure in the future. Like Julia, Millennials who spend years living with their parents may be better able to pay off their student loans, become debt-free, and maybe even save enough to purchase their own homes. Taking the time now to figure out where they want to go in life could help Millennials avoid a life course disruption years down the line, when it could interrupt their own children' lives. In short, Millennials may be setting themselves up to be great parents.

CHAPTER TWO

Plans:
How Women Make, Break, and
Follow Through on Them

In season one of hit TV series *Jane the Virgin*, Petra has to make a choice. To artificially inseminate herself or not—that is the question. The show's narrator explains her decision-making process: "Last night, after stealing her ex-husband's sperm, Petra did what any reasonable person would do: she drunk-dialed her mother. After being hung up on three times … Petra decided to make a pro/con list." She drunkenly scribbles:

Cons
pregnant
baby
motherhood
maternity clothes
seem like a psychopath

As for the pros, the narrator emphasizes, "There was just the one: Rafael." If she gets pregnant with her ex's child, Petra thinks she can win him back. And with that, all the cons melt away—they literally dissolve off the TV screen. Petra gazes—through beer goggles—at Rafael's sperm sample. And just like that, you can tell she's made up her mind.

There are plenty of reasons not to compare fiction with reality. But suspend your disbelief for the moment; I'll talk more about that later. For now, think about how Petra went about making this decision. She resorted to a list: a clear-cut, logical chart that let her weigh the pros and cons. We often (mistakenly) think that humans make decisions this way. Even researchers are guilty of assuming that choices are the products of cost-benefit analyses.[78] When it comes to WiSK decisions, we think women operate like Petra. We think they calculatedly look at things like child care, maternity leave, income, housing, and then decide to want, start, and keep babies only if it's to their advantage, all of these things considered. The implication is that women choose to have a child—or choose to avoid it— by rationally weighing the pros and cons.[79]

That's plainly untrue. Just look at how well Petra's pro/con list worked. Despite having a single pro and several very valid cons, she still wants, starts, and—spoiler alert!—keeps her twin baby girls.

Petra's decision making is clearly ridiculous, so here are some more realistic examples. The first is teen mothers. Most of these girls don't *choose* to get pregnant. They certainly didn't do a cost-benefit analysis and conclude that having a baby would be in their best interest. Though typically dismissed as irresponsible, teen moms aren't the only ones making (economically) irrational choices. It costs an average of $253,954 to raise a child to age 18 in Canada.[80] That's $1,366 a month before they even start university. Not every Canadian can afford that. But clearly, not all Canadians are thinking about money when they make WiSK decisions. If we did, only a narrow slice of the population would ever get pregnant.

So, human decisions aren't always calculated—especially when family, love, and sex are involved. If we don't weigh pros and cons, how *do* we make choices? The answer to that question is what this chapter's all about.

Questions you'll get answers to:

▶ *How do different women, with different characteristics and resources, make WiSK decisions?*

▶ *What factors do women consider when making WiSK decisions?*

▶ *Do WiSK decisions change when people couple up? How do our partners' plans influence our own?*

▶ *Do most women act on the plans they make when young? Or do many change their minds, and abandon their earlier decisions?*

The Factor Funnel

Jane—the star of the same show that features Petra's hilarious plan to win Rafael back—also has to make a choice. She's been accidentally artificially inseminated with none other than Rafael's sperm. Now carrying the baby of a stranger (who happens to own the hotel where she works, and whom she happens to have a fleeting romantic history with), Jane must decide if she's going to keep the baby. Unlike Petra, Jane doesn't make a list, or weigh her pros and cons. But for the sake of simplifying the show's complicated plot, here's a list of the main factors Jane considers:

1. Jane's boyfriend proposes right before she tells him she's pregnant with another man's child. Michael begs her not to have the baby, so they can start their life together.

2. Rafael is a cancer survivor who will never be able to have a biological child if Jane doesn't have this baby (or so we believe at this point in the telenovela). His sister—who also happens to be the doctor responsible for the accidental artificial insemination—begs Jane to keep the baby, telling her it was his last sperm sample.

3. Rafael assures Jane that he and his wife would "take it." So, she would be giving the baby to a loving family that wants it, not worrying about finding adoptive parents.

4. Jane herself is the product of an unplanned pregnancy, and she desperately wants to avoid following in her mom's footsteps and having her carefully planned life derailed.

5. Jane's Abuela urges her to keep the baby, assuring her that it "will be the best part of your life."

6. Jane's mom emphasizes that the choice is entirely up to her. Xo even picks up a prescription for an oral abortion.

Jane contemplates these—and many other—factors within the very first episode. As she sits on the bus, we see what's going on inside her head: a montage of all the players, pithily stating their opinions. We see Xo, Rafael, Michael, and Abuela swirling around in Jane's brain. Out of the chaotic montage, full of contradictory views, Jane decides: "I'm having the baby."

Though the decision itself is unconventional, the process Jane went through to make it is realistic. Decision making works like a funnel. Multiple considerations go in to the funnel through its wide opening at the top. They all swirl around together, before one end result comes out the bottom.

WiSK decisions are no exception. The decisions to want, start, and keep a baby emerge from the bottom of a funnel with a huge mouth, where countless factors have intermingled to produce the end result.

What are those factors? In this chapter, I look at three: government policies, family, and personal circumstances. We'll see how women funnel these considerations together, and end up with their WiSK decisions. And we'll see how these funnels differ for different women—that is, for women of different ages, races, educational levels, and so on.

Government policies come first because they are at the widest point of the funnel for most women. They set the stage for women's decision making in very broad terms, but they are not top of mind as women make WiSK decisions. Next comes family. Women—and men—think more consciously about their experiences with their existing family members when making WiSK decisions. As we will see, they ask themselves how they might imitate the positive aspects of family life they enjoyed growing up. And they ask how they might avoid the negative aspects. Finally, I drill down to the deeply personal. Living arrangements, finding a partner, career goals, and other individual preferences are at the forefront of WiSK decision making. So, let's start at the broad mouth of the factor funnel and move down to its narrow end, tracing WiSK decision making patterns as we go.

Part I: Government Policies
Pro-Baby Incentives
In the late 1980s, Quebec implemented a game-changing policy (or so we thought at the time). The Allowance for Newborn Children (ANC) was a non-taxable baby bonus. It was given to all legal Quebec residents who had a child between May 1988 and September 1997. The ANC was just one thing the government was doing to try to encourage more people to have babies.[81]

Common sense predicted that, with this new bonus enticing people to have kids … well, more people would have kids. But in the 1980s and '90s, fertility rates in Quebec stayed similar to, or even dipped below, those across Canada.[82] We certainly didn't see a Quebecois baby boom in response to the ANC.

This is a huge discovery. We tend to point the finger at family policies—or a lack thereof—when we talk about lagging fertility rates.[83] And governments can be quick to jump on the baby-bonus bandwagon to try to show their constituents they're taking action to help families.[84] But as the ANC showed, the relationship between family policies and WiSK decisions is not straightforward.

In theory, cash benefits, subsidized childcare, and long, paid parental leave should encourage women to have children.[85] And in theory, the absence of these supports should discourage childbearing. But this common-sense rationale is simplistic. Government-mandated family policies are the last thing you think about when making WiSK decisions. Research shows that many parents do indeed accept and benefit from policies like baby bonuses. But few take these policies into consideration when deciding whether or not to have a child.[86]

Instead, government policies are just one variable that gets thrown into women's WiSK decision funnel, usually unconsciously. These policies swirl around in that funnel, along with a bunch of personal considerations like:

- the amount of money or time off a woman will receive if she accepts a benefit like paid leave;
- the conditions she needs to meet to claim a given benefit, such as the number of hours she would need to work before getting paid leave;
- the opportunities and money she has access to, regardless of the policy; and
- the stigma attached to receiving certain benefits.

These considerations determine whether women will even consider accepting benefits.[87] And because so many variables are interacting—swirling around together in the funnel—it's difficult to say which ones influence WiSK decisions most.[88] It's also difficult to disentangle these policy-related factors from others, like career goals.

Studies looking at policies across different countries help explain why. Sometimes, those studies show higher fertility rates in countries offering more generous benefits, and lower fertility rates in countries offering less. But countries offering more generous family benefits are usually the ones with better social safety nets. Beyond things like cash baby bonuses and paid parental leave, they may also provide more generous low-income supports. Parents in these countries may consider income top-ups more seriously during their WiSK deliberations than they do one-time baby bonuses. We have no way of knowing whether they have kids because they know their income will be supplemented, or because they know they'll get the bonus. And on the other hand, many countries offer minimal support for childbearing, but have high fertility rates nonetheless.

What we do know is that some women use family policies more than others. Middle-earning women benefit most. But for high- and low-income earners, pro-natal policies don't make much of a difference.

First, consider high-income earners. Some researchers assume these couples will have more children. With more money, they don't have to worry about being able to provide for their children. But in modern societies, high-earning couples *do not* have a lot of children, on average.[89] That's because people who earn more correctly expect their children to cost more (Gauthier 2007). They anticipate signing their children up for costly extracurricular activities like ballet and hockey lessons; paying for private school or private tutors; and supporting their children through university and even graduate school. Providing a high standard of living for a child is much more costly than meeting their basic needs.

Family policies do little to change this picture. For people earning high incomes, a cash benefit may not make a difference. It may be so small, relative to their overall incomes, that it doesn't even go in to their WiSK decision funnel.

Now, consider people earning low incomes. A cash benefit

may not make a difference for them either. They may feel as though they'll never be financially stable enough to comfortably support children. But plenty of low-income earners have children nevertheless.

The same is true when it comes to parental leave. Low-income earners might not be able to live off of the reduced wages they'd earn on leave. And high-income earners may worry about keeping up with their competitors after months away from the job. Once again, middle-earning women are the ones who find this incentive in their WiSK decision funnel.

In sum, the small relationship researchers sometimes find between family policies and fertility is an association at best; we can't show these policies *cause* couples to have children.[90] Also, the association is observed mainly in certain segments of the population. As we have seen, middle-earning women are most responsive to these policies, compared with low- and high-income earners. They likely do not cause them to have more children than they intended—the explicit hope of many pro-natal policies.

In fact, these policies do less to influence our personal decisions than our broad views as a society. Policies don't just affect the way parents see the economic costs of having children. They also affect how people see families.[91] For example, laws that permit long, generous parental leaves show that our society values families and children very much. Such laws make childbearing and child care appear professionally and socially acceptable. That's why these policies appear, for most women, at the very broad opening of the WiSK factor funnel. They merely set the stage for those decisions, but they do not play a starring role.

Child Care
To Have It All, women need support. Like I mentioned in the last chapter, we don't live in an equal society. In most households, women do more housework and child care than men. Evening things out is the first step towards supporting those women who want to enjoy careers, relationships, *and* motherhood.

Affordable, accessible child care is typically offered as a solution. We often assume that mothers who can use child care services can continue working.[92] We also assume that child care allows women to have as many children as they want, at whatever age they want.[93]

In reality, though, many couples don't or can't use child care services. Sometimes, our personal values and beliefs get in the way. Many believe women should care for their own children.[94] In other cases, women's husbands may support their careers, but refuse to change their own work schedules. If her husband refuses to pitch in, a mother doesn't really have a choice. She may have to leave her work—temporarily or permanently—or reduce her hours.[95]

In other cases still, it's our child care system that's falling short. Women have joined the workforce at a rapid rate over the past several decades, but child care services haven't kept pace.[96] Waitlists for child care can take years. Child care is also expensive, especially when two or more children need care. Sometimes, these costs outstrip what women can earn working, making it more financially sensible for them to stay home.

But even in places like Scandinavia, where child care is widely available and affordable, problems still arise. Having the option to send your hypothetical child to day care sometime in the future isn't enough to push people to start a family. And not having that option isn't enough to deter others. So, much like pro-natal policies, child care does little to directly influence women's WiSK decisions.[97]

Make no mistake: child care can indeed help women Have It All. Many women now get to enjoy better-balanced work and family lives, thanks to affordable, accessible child care services. But few—if any—of those women made their WiSK decisions with child care at the top of their minds. Like pro-natal policies, child care is at the very widest part of the funnel: at the back of women's minds, perhaps, reminding them that the family is such an important institution, the state backs it.

Part II: Family

We all learn how to think about marriage and family when we're young.[98] Based on our parents' interactions, couples' behaviour on TV, marriages and divorces broadcast on social media, and other depictions of relationships, we develop ideas of what coupledom is supposed to look like. These attitudes, which start forming when we're kids, remain more or less stable throughout life.

Parental Structure

Family structures—and rearrangements of those structures—are perhaps the biggest influence. Your childhood living arrangements often have implications for your own WiSK decisions.[99] Most directly, women typically know about their mothers' history of marriage and childbearing. That knowledge shapes their understanding of what's "normal." In turn, norms learned from our mother's behaviour influence the WiSK decisions we make ourselves.

How does this play out? Generally, people tend to mirror their parents' behaviour or do the exact opposite. The quality of relationship between parents and their children determines which option you take.[100] Children who are close with their parents are likely to mirror their parents' behavior. On the other hand, children with distant, tense relationships with their parents are likely to do opposite.

For example, consider a woman whose parents married young, had kids early, stayed together, and raised a tight-knit family. That woman may follow the example her parents set, getting married early, but waiting to have kids until she does. She has grown up in a positive home environment that she might want to emulate. On the other hand, a woman who endured her parents' nasty divorce may vow to avoid subjecting her own children to the same hardships. She might be more cautious about getting into a serious relationship. She might marry later than average, to reassure herself she's found the "right person." And she may avoid having children of her own.

So, kids tend to learn from their parents. Childhood experiences influence women's timing and ordering preferences: how old they want to be when they do certain things, and the order in which they want to do them.[101] As mentioned in the previous chapter, the traditional ordering of standard life course events is:

1. Move out of your parents' house.
2. Get married.
3. Have children.

Ordering and timing preferences vary, based on the type of household women grew up in.

Two-Parent Households

Children who grew up with two parents are most likely to follow the traditional ordering: they leave the nest, get married, then have children. They are less likely to have an "early" birth, before age 20. This is in part because children who are raised in dual-parent households get more supervision.[102] One of the two parents is more likely to be around, making it more difficult for the child to pursue romantic relationships.

Divorced Parents

Children whose parents divorced are more cautious about marriage. They want to avoid subjecting their children to the painful experiences they themselves endured. As such, they marry later than average, in an effort to make themselves feel as confident as possible in their relationship. They are more likely to cohabit before marrying, as a "test" of the relationship I described in the last chapter.[103]

When divorced or widowed parents remarry, their children often struggle to connect with the new stepparent. The child-stepparent relationship may be strained, often because the child resents the new spouse for trying to take their biological parent's "place." Or, the child may feel that their presence—a reminder of the deceased or divorced spouse—has a negative impact on the stepparent's or both parents' relationship satisfaction. Either way, children from "broken homes" are more likely to leave the parental nest early, likely in an effort to gain distance from the stepparent. But these young adults may be especially *unlikely* to have children early. They know having a baby would bring certain (and heavy) costs. For example, they might need to rely on their parent and stepparent to help care for it, which would force them to spend more time with the people they were trying to avoid. So, girls who think that having a child would carry negative costs may be especially careful with contraception, or especially willing to have an abortion.

That said, some daughters of divorced parents are at risk for young, single motherhood. When their families are disrupted in this way, some young adults may come to feel like they have little control over what happens to them.[104] Careful planning for their future may, in turn, seem futile. Because they think their circumstances are beyond their control, these youth may make important decisions lightly. For example, they may not use contraceptives consistently. Or, they may be more willing to have a baby they conceived accidentally, not taking into account how it may interrupt their educational or occupational plans. Finally, in their effort to cope, these girls may come to rely more on their own romantic partnerships in a search for emotional support and stability. This may lead them to get more serious with their partners, by marrying and/or having a child.

Single Parents

Lastly, girls raised by single mothers are more likely to become single mothers themselves. And girls raised by teen mothers are 51 percent more likely to become teen mothers themselves.[105]

As mentioned above, girls with single parents may not spend as much time under direct parental supervision. Romantic (and sexual) attention may seem even more important to girls whose parent isn't around a lot, or doesn't have a strong, supportive relationship with their child. As a result, they're more likely to start dating and having sex at younger-than-average ages, as they seek attention, affection, and love from people other than their family members. In turn, they're more likely to get accidentally pregnant than others. What's more, these girls grew up with a single parent as their role model, witnessing how single parenthood can be *made* to work. If they get pregnant as teens, these girls are more likely to keep the baby because they don't think they need the help of the father to take care of it.

Others see early motherhood as a way to demonstrate their maturity. Girls born into poor, racialized families have slimmer-than-average chances of going to a good school, or getting a good job. Those who live in isolated, low-income areas are even more likely to think their opportunities are limited, and that motherhood is one of the only roles available to women.[106] They recognize they won't be able to have a rewarding career, so they settle for a role that's within their reach: motherhood.

All of this is to say that single motherhood and even teen pregnancy aren't always accidental. Nor are they the result of young adults' lazy reluctance to use contraceptives. Rather, some girls deliberately choose motherhood if they think they don't have any other means of achieving adulthood. In their eyes, getting pregnant seems like an escape from childhood in their parents' home, where they're seen as powerless non-adults.

The unlikelihood of interracial relationships also plays a role. When they do marry, black women typically marry black men. However, black men are subject to educational and occupational disadvantages that have led to higher un- and under-employment rates. Black men, especially in the United States, are also more likely to be incarcerated. This makes them physically unavailable for marriage and also reduces their chances of securing steady employment after their release. So, in assessing their marital prospects, black women may come to think they would be better off remaining unmarried—even if they get pregnant or already have a child—than marrying a man who cannot help support their family. This explains why many black women never marry or marry at later ages than white women,[107] and why many single-parent households are run by black women.

All of that said, being raised by a single parent doesn't mean you're fated to become one too. Many women are painfully aware of their single mother's struggle: having to work multiple jobs to make ends meet, shouldering all child care and household responsibilities alone, not having emotional support from a partner, and so on. Growing up with a single parent may motivate some women to avoid the same circumstances for themselves and their own children.[108]

Family Religion

Religious affiliation by itself doesn't tell us much about women's WiSK decisions. Plenty of rebellious teens shun the religious beliefs their parents live by. Just because a girl was raised Catholic, for example, doesn't mean she'll abstain from sex until marriage. More important is "religiosity": the degree to which people genuinely endorse their religion.

Very religious people tend to hold strong views about sex, marriage, childbearing, and parenthood, especially in the United States.[109] It is hard for children and teens to form their own opinions when their parents encourage adherence to the views spelled out in their religion. As such, youth who become as religious as their parents may be less willing to:

- have pre-marital sex,
- live with their partners before marrying them, and
- abort unplanned pregnancies.[110]

And they may believe more strongly that:

- marriage is sacred,
- birth control is unacceptable,
- large families with lots of kids are desirable, and
- women should be the main caregivers for those kids.[111]

Consider cohabitation. For religious people, moving in with a partner is a public declaration that that couple is no longer abstaining from sex. Young religious people may therefore avoid cohabiting out of fear that they'll attract negative judgments from their community. Sometimes, a young person's parents may keep her from moving in with her partner because they care what their communities think about their family, even if they are not religious themselves. In the end, this means Catholics leave the nest later than average, because they wait until they're married to do so.

Some of this is due to geographic location. Women who live in rural areas are more likely to get married earlier. People in rural areas tend to hold on to traditional family values. Rural regions also present few educational and work opportunities for women, thereby offering women few alternatives to marriage and motherhood.

Overall, women who are more religious—regardless of the specific religion they belong to—are more likely to want kids, start them only after they're married, and keep any unplanned pregnancies. They typically abstain from pre-marital sex, and usually do not cohabit before marriage.[112] Once married, they are unlikely to use contraceptives, and (unsurprisingly) they have many children. Finally, highly religious women are at a lower risk of divorce than non-religious women.

All of that said, religion has played less and less of a role in determining fertility trends in recent years. Religious and non-religious groups are becoming more alike in terms of their childbearing desires and behaviours.[113]

Parental Education and Socioeconomic Status

Parents pass more than family values along to their children. Just as girls learn what marriage is "supposed" to look like by watching their parents, they also learn the importance of education from their parents.[114] Girls with college-educated, stably employed parents recognize the value of a higher education: they see how education has helped their parents succeed in life. As a result, they're likely to want to go to college too.

How does this impact their WiSK decisions? First, these young women are more likely to move out of their parents' home in their late teenage years, and into a dorm or apartment to go to school. And once they finish school, they usually hope to get a job that pays well enough to let them continue living independently. Given their background, children of educated parents are often *able* to move out when they want to, at younger ages, because their parents may support them financially if they need help. Usually, educated parents are happy to help— so long as their kids aren't moving out to get married. These parents support independence, and discourage their children from letting marriage and kids interrupt their education and career. Often, kids with highly educated parents are on the same page. They *want* to finish school and start working before beginning a family, because they've been taught to value this standard life course. And, as I will discuss shortly, women who live independently enjoy a taste of freedom that often leads them to postpone marriage and childbearing.

By contrast, women are unlikely to live independently when they're born into low-income families, and have parents with less than a high school education. They have slim chances of going to a good school, or getting a good job. So on the whole, they leave the nest later than average. In turn, daughters of less-educated parents are more likely to get married and have their first child before moving out of their parents' home. These women might have a similar mindset as the daughters of single mothers described above. They might not see a university degree, full time job, or even marriage as indicators of adulthood. Recognizing they won't be able to attain these things, they settle for a role that's within their reach: motherhood.

As mentioned above, these patterns reflect ideas about adulthood and its attainability: less privileged women may view parenthood as the only viable path into adulthood, in the absence of other educational or employment opportunities. In comparison, privileged women are more interested in attaining an education and a career; they have opportunities, and they know it. With higher hopes for their future, privileged women have an incentive to hold off on marriage and childbearing.

Race

Women of different races tend to get married and have kids at different ages and life stages. The most common ordering of life course events among black, Hispanic, and white people is:

- Black: give birth, get married, move out;
- Hispanic: get married, give birth, move out;
- White: move out, get married, give birth.[115]

Sometimes this has to do with overlaps between education, racialization, and socioeconomic status. In the United States even more than in Canada, people of different races are born with unequal life chances. That is, they have different chances to get an education and compete for good jobs. Because of inherited class differences, white children are more likely to go to university and secure a stable job than black children. So, white children are more likely to come from the educated, higher socioeconomic-status families described above. And black and Hispanic children are more likely to come from the less educated, lower socioeconomic-status families. As such, Black and Hispanic parents are less likely to expect their children to live independently before marrying than white parents. (This has been attributed, without empirical evidence, to their more "traditional" values.) So, these youth leave the nest later than white people. Because they leave the nest later, they are more likely to have their first child while still living at home.

Part III: Personal Circumstances

At the very bottom of the WiSK factor funnel are our conscious thought processes. These are the active deliberations we have with ourselves and others over whether we want kids, and when.

There are at least two ways young women consciously think about children as part of their life plan. The first way is uncertain and the second is assured.

First, some women think about having children only occasionally and in vague terms. They aren't sure if they want children at all. If they do, they have a checklist of things that need to happen first. For example, they want to finish school, then get a job, then find a suitable partner, then find a home with that partner. Only when all of these prerequisites have been fulfilled would this first "type" of woman entertain the idea of having a child.

Second, some women know, from an early age, that they absolutely want children. To reach that goal, they develop a schedule. They consider what checklist items need to be taken care of immediately before giving birth, what items need to be attained before that, and so on. Thinking backwards from the goal of giving birth, they may reason that they want to share a home with their partner first; but to share that home, they would need to find a suitable partner; to have found that partner, they would need to date; and to be an attractive date, they would have to get an education and a good job.

No matter which camp they fall into, all women start off single, at some point in their lives.

The Single Years

Many of the emerging adults I discussed in the last chapter experiment with living arrangements. Be it a college dormitory, basement bachelor pad, or 3-bedroom flat split between roommates, many 18-to-20-somethings live away from their parents. These living arrangements both facilitate sex and provide an incentive *not* to get pregnant.

Consider, for example, a college freshman who's never lived away from home before. She'll take advantage of her new freedom. Without her parents' surveillance, she's able to date and have sex much more easily. For slightly older young women, living away from mom and dad may make relationships feel more serious. These women might start mirroring the behaviour of married couples by sleeping at each other's houses, making meals together, and so on. In both instances, sexual contact increases, so the risk of becoming pregnant does too.

However, among these adults, the *desire* to have a baby may dip lower than ever before. They're enjoying their first taste of freedom, and won't want to give it up to become a mother. These women often want to maintain their newly acquired independence, which a baby—and all of its related expenses and responsibilities—would threaten. For these reasons, women living independently for the first time may be more careful about using contraceptives—or more open to having an abortion—than women still living with their parents.

This is all part of what researchers call a "role hiatus". These women are, often just briefly, not defined by their roles as daughters, wives, and mothers. They don't need to live up to the rules their parents set for them while they were living at home as children. They're also free from the responsibilities they will assume as parents and homemakers.

A role hiatus may change the way a young woman plans her life. Without daughterly/wifely/motherly responsibilities, she can focus on school and work. As a result, she may come to like the idea of a career more than that of motherhood. Unless her parents are helping her, this young woman will also be using her own earnings to support herself. She recognizes the value of her work, develops a strong sense of responsibility, and understands what her independence is worth. In turn, she may also develop more liberal ideas about families, coming to believe, for example, that:

- having fewer children is desirable;
- husbands and wives should share the responsibility of caring for their children more or less equally; and
- it's acceptable for mothers to work outside of the home.

With these values, women who live independently might opt to stay single for longer. After all, they don't *need* to depend on a man to be the breadwinner or to help out around the house.[116] In this sense, marriage is no longer "necessary" for them, as it was for women in the past who received little education and were unable to get a well-paying job.[117] Instead, marriage might seem costly—an infringement on the independence they earned by setting out on their own.

Emerging adults' love of independence is part of the reason why many women are marrying later. It's common today for people to resolve to put off marriage until they've accomplished whatever they set out in life to do.[118] For some, this means establishing a successful career, while for others, it means travelling the world, or buying a house. For a majority, financial stability is a prerequisite for marriage.[119] From this perspective, marriage and childbearing are signs: symbols people use to show they've fulfilled other life goals.[120]

When or if they do decide to settle down with a partner, these educated, independent women are freer to choose their spouses based on things like romantic attraction and compatibility. At least in theory, couples who get together by choice rather than necessity tend to stay together long-term. They're often more satisfied in their relationship, and raise children based on shared values.

So, taking a role hiatus makes women more likely to delay marriage and childbearing; to get more education and a better job; and to develop more egalitarian views on marital roles.[121] Conversely, having children before leaving home makes women more likely to get married early; have more children overall; get less education; and get a low-paying, precarious job, or no job at all.

Finally, women who take a role hiatus when they're young may be more satisfied with motherhood when (or if) they do decide to have children. Taking time to live by herself may better prepare a woman to live with a partner, and eventually, with children. Independent living teaches her how to support and care for *herself* before she has to try to care for others. When these women do have children, they've already got their own needs and wants figured out, instead of trying to learn how to care for themselves, their husbands, and their children all at once.

The Hunt for a Partner

When it comes to the checklist of life events that need to happen before you have your first child, the most important is finding a suitable partner. Besides things like chemistry and love that we can't reliably measure, plenty of social factors predict who and when a woman is most likely to marry. Let's start with who.

People's spouse selection is affected by the size and composition of their social networks: their family, friends, and acquaintances. People associate with one another—and, from this pool of acquaintances, select potential dates—based on the principle of homogamy.[122] In short, homogamy describes social similarity. People are more likely to date others with similar personal characteristics, including political attitudes, lifestyles, values, appearances, and ethnicities.[123] They are especially likely to date—and marry—people with similar levels of education, from similar social classes. Opposites may attract initially, but they're rarely able to sustain stable, long-term relationships.

Homogamous relations develop for at least two reasons: preference and exposure. First, people prefer to interact with others like them. Sharply diverging views, beliefs, and values cause conflict. But shared experiences and preferences promote easy conversation and close bonds. So, people tend to spend their time, when possible, with others like themselves. And they tend to see these people as attractive mates.[124]

Second, socially similar people are thrown together in many different settings: classrooms, workplaces, neighborhoods, gyms, bars, and so on. That means these socially similar people are likely to meet, spend time together, and develop emotional bonds. Exposure thus promotes the meeting of similar people, while preference sustains their relationship in the long term.

Once homogamy has helped a woman find someone suitable, how long will it take for them to get married? In terms of timing, a person's family of origin is the most important variable that may either propel her into or hold her back from marriage.

Certain events "trigger" or delay marriage. Triggers include watching other family members—siblings, parents, aunts, uncles, grandparents, and so on—get married, divorce, have children of their own, retire, move elsewhere, or pass away.[125] For many, these events are "disruptive": they disturb the day-to-day monotony we all grow used to. People who experience these events commonly try to restore order and balance in their lives. Marriage, representing stability, long-term commitment, and a predictable future, may be seen as a way to get back "on track" in the life course.

This is especially true for people who have close family relations.[126] The death of a great aunt you've never met probably won't push you to make a life-altering decision. But the death of your mother might. Birth order also plays a role here. Oldest children and only children are often closest with their families. When these people experience such disruptive events, they are more likely than other children to respond by marrying. Such a response is also more common among women than men.

People of different ages may have different reasons for responding to disruptive life events in the way they do, but they respond the same: by making stabilizing, balance-restoring changes. A teenager who watches her parents split up may yearn to get married ASAP because she's clinging to her long-term boyfriend for some stability. And a 40-something bohemian whose brother unexpectedly passes away may likewise suddenly hear the siren call of stable married life.

So, the random timing of disruptive events may cause a life course to take an unplanned turn. Equally important are socio-economic conditions and ambitions. Alone or in combination with a disruptive event, your parents' income may cause you to marry "early," "on time," or "late." (By way of a shorthand definition, women who marry "early" are in their teens; those who marry "on time" are in their twenties; and those who marry "late" are in their thirties. Like generations, these timelines are loosely defined, and vary across different societies. Toronto women who get engaged at age 27 aren't seen as "late" marry-ers. But unmarried 27-year-olds in some rural, conservative Ontario neighbourhoods may be seen as getting on in years.)

Early marrying women tend to come from lower-income families with low educational and occupational aspirations. Women with higher educational or occupational plans are more likely to marry "on time" or "late," especially if they come from middle or upper income families. As discussed in the previous chapter, many women prefer to finish school and begin their career before marrying.[127] Thus, highly educated, occupationally ambitious women who enjoy an income cushion at home marry later.

So, who and when you marry isn't just about feeling "ready," or even finding someone with a personality that meshes with yours. Finding a life partner is also about being in the right place at the right time. Women who want a financially stable husband may never find one if they aren't on the college campuses or in the workplaces where such men spend most of their time. Equally, couples who have been happily dating for years may never take the next step and get married if they aren't pushed to do so by a disruptive event.

Making WiSK Decisions as One Half of a Couple
Plenty of people love a good romance. The wild popularity of shows like *Jane the Virgin* and *The Bachelor* indicates that our culture is obsessed with love. We believe in love at first sight, think love can conquer all, and swipe endlessly through our

phones, looking for the "soul mate" we're meant to spend forever with.

Real life isn't a rom com, though. In reality, it's almost always the principle of homogamy—not love—that comes out on top. People prove, time and again, that some differences are too big to set aside. One of those insurmountable differences, for many couples, is WiSK decisions.

Thanks to homogamy, we tend to settle down with people who share our values. That means, most of the time, people who end up together have similar—though not identical—plans for their future.

Usually, people who value family and children end up together. These couples typically have similar WiSK plans: they both want kids, and just need to agree on exactly how many, and when to start having them.[128] On the other hand, people who don't want kids often end up together. They share common values, too: perhaps they deeply value their careers, or want to put their relationship first. One study[129] found couples resolutely agreed on this front: of *all* the women surveyed who said they wanted to stay child free, not a single one of their male partners disagreed and said they were planning to have a child.

Sometimes, this agreement is the result of compromise.[130] As we've seen, WiSK decisions are far from black and white. Plenty of women are unsure about whether they want kids, when, or how many. Falling in love with someone who absolutely wants a family can be enough to push these undecided women to go along for the ride. Or, settling down with someone who absolutely does not want children can push them to stay child free.

Your partner's wishes are thus another factor in your WiSK decision funnel. When they get thrown into the mix, you need to reconsider the plans you made before meeting them.[131]

That said, long-term matches between someone who definitely wants kids and someone who definitely does not are far less common. When there's no room for compromise on this important front, the strain on a relationship may be too great. Typically, one of two things will happen. One: the conflicted couple may break up, having realized they want different things in life. Or two: one of them will sacrifice their original WiSK plans. In the latter case, who is most likely to come out on top—which partner will win the other one over?

We sometimes fall into the trap of assuming that these decisions are all about power, and which half of the couple has more of it.[132] In patriarchal societies, for example, we might expect men to get their way more often than women. In reality though, it's not so much about gender or power as it is about social context.[133] In most relationships, neither women nor men have the final say. Rather, the person with the more average WiSK plans will likely get their way. That's because social norms exert a powerful influence over our WiSK decisions— something I talk about in great detail in chapters four and five of this book.

For now, consider an example. Say Laura wants four kids, but her partner Jordan just wants two. Because two-child families are the norm in our society, the couple will feel like Jordan's got the whole world behind him. Eventually, Laura will probably be the one to compromise, adjust her original WiSK plans, and have just two or maybe three kids: an average family size that's more widely supported in our culture.

Because they depend on social context, these WiSK negotiations can go different ways depending where you live. In our society, small preferences tend to dominate.[134] That means the person who wants fewer—if any—kids usually wins. So, for example, a single woman may plan to have two kids. But if she partners up with a man who doesn't want any kids at all, chances are the couple will stay childfree (if they stay together).[135] Things work differently in different societies, though. In less-developed regions, where large families are valued, the spouse with the larger preference may dominate.[136]

Opportunities or Opportunity Costs?

Work is one of the most important, frequently surfacing questions swirling around in the WiSK factor funnel. Depending on their socioeconomic background, women may see having a child as an opportunity, or as a barrier that will force them to give up opportunities. Women with lots of education and good job opportunities may see having a child as an "opportunity cost": something they do at the expense of their other options, including a rewarding career.[137] But for women with little or no education and poor job prospects, having a child may look like a great opportunity: one that will help them solidify their adult status and their partner's commitment.

As a woman's level of education and earning potential increases, so does the opportunity cost of having children.[138] Opportunity costs include three things. The first is lost wages. When a woman takes time off work or quits her job to have children, she no longer earns money from that job. Her household income drops as a result. The second is reduced or lost career prospects. To accommodate her new childcare responsibilities, a new mother may no longer be able to work full time. To work fewer hours, or have greater flexibility at work, she may have to accept a lower-paying or less-rewarding job. She may not even be able to work at all, and have to give up her career altogether.[139]

The third cost is a reduced return on her educational investment. This mainly applies to women who needed to gain lots of education and/or experience to find work in their field. Even if they get paid maternity leave, these women will fall "behind" in their fields while women still at work forge ahead. When they return, these new mothers won't be at the top of the list for a promotion or raise; they'll be expected to spend time catching up. In this sense, highly-educated mothers enjoy less of a return on their investments in education, training, and work experience than they would if they hadn't interrupted their careers to have children.

In sum, opportunity costs help explain how education is connected to the age at which a woman becomes a mother. Women who only get a high school diploma can easily have children at younger ages, often in their early or mid-twenties. They may plan to have children while young because they see few alternatives to motherhood, as discussed above. And even if they didn't plan for it, these women didn't have big educational or career aspirations to be derailed anyway.

By contrast, more highly educated women get married and have children later.[140] Busy with school until their mid-twenties, they put off their family plans until they've completed their degree(s).[141] Consider a study that compared two groups of married women: one group that was enrolled in school and another that was not. Those who were still enrolled were 41 percent less likely to have a child at home than the married women who were not in school.[142]

Final Thoughts

Today, fertility rates consistently fall below people's earlier-stated ideals. When asked in surveys or polls how many children they intend to have, many young adult women say two.[143] But research also shows that these intentions are often not realized. Most women today have fewer children than they originally plan to.[144]

This is because family size—the number of children a woman bears—has more to do with other life plans than with the number of children someone dreamt up while still a girl. Life doesn't always turn out the way we hope it will, and the WiSK plans we make for ourselves while young shape our futures only to a limited extent.

In this sense, the best indicator of people's fertility intentions is not the number of children they say they are going to have. Instead, it is their stated commitment to other life goals, such as higher education and a professional career. People who plan to complete a lot of post-secondary education usually go on to do at least some university. And people with high educational aspirations usually plan, from a young age, to get married after completing their education. So, a strong childhood commitment to education often translates into higher educational attainment and prevents other life goals—like having children—from interrupting those plans.

For this reason, as women's education and employment attainments increase, women revise their original WiSK decisions. They change their plans to have fewer children, starting at older ages. In other words, some women want more children than they even *plan* to have—let alone give birth to—because of the current tensions between motherhood and paid employment. So women have fewer children than they consider ideal because they come up against real-life barriers, such as the high costs of having children, and the inability to balance work with motherhood.[145]

Sociologists use "role incompatibility theory" to describe this tension.[146] Going to school, working, and raising children all take time and energy. In turn, women experience a "strain" between all the roles they are trying to fill: student, employee, and mother. Women who choose to pursue educational and career goals may not be able to fit children into the mix, and adjust or abandon their WiSK decisions accordingly.

Recall rational choice theory, discussed at the beginning of this chapter. Its main assumption is that people make WiSK decisions after weighing their pros and cons.[147] The problem, we now see, is that most people don't know much about the pros and cons of having a child until they have one.

In reality, people always make decisions based on imperfect, incomplete information and (often faulty) assumptions about the future.[148] These assumptions are based on people's current social circumstances: what they have witnessed among their friends, family, acquaintances, TV shows, books, films, and so on. For example, people whose own mothers, female relatives, and female friends quit their jobs to raise children may come to think that mothers don't have time for paid work on top of mothering. Surrounded by stay-at-home mothers, career-driven women may think they have to choose between work and family.

Similarly, in social circles where newborns are routinely showered with expensive toys, clothes, strollers, cribs, and other accessories, the cost of raising a child may seem overwhelming. That can make low-income earners believe they can't afford a family. What shapes a woman's decision to have a child is how much she *thinks* it costs, the proportion of her income she's willing to devote to those costs, and what she believes she'd have to give up to devote that much money to her child. The actual cost of raising a child is irrelevant.

Often, information is also incomplete in the sense that no

one can foresee what their lives will be like in the future. We all make educated guesses, based on our present job stability and income, about what we'll earn in the coming years.[149] We think about whether we'll make enough to support a two-year-old baby, for example; or, whether we'll be enjoying our career so much, we won't want to give it up to take care of that baby. Some of these guesses are more accurate than others. For example, a lawyer may be better able to predict her earning trajectory than a bartender. High uncertainty about these things may deter people from even planning to have children; or if things fail to unfold as predicted, people may change their original intentions.

When people make important decisions based on imperfect, incomplete information, there are two consequences. First, both they and their children may wind up deeply disappointed and, sometimes, even harmed. I address this concern in the final chapter of this book. Second, after having one child, and by doing so gaining more accurate information about the consequences, women may adjust their long-term family plans.

Few decisions in life are as important and frequently discussed as WiSK decisions. But despite their life-altering potential, WiSK decisions are also frequently changed or abandoned. The factor funnel helps explain why. These decisions are not made using Petra's straightforward pro/con list. Rather, they are constantly being renegotiated, based on a constantly changing list of factors being poured into the funnel. As we grow up, we learn about the importance of marriage and childbearing from the two institutions at the very top of the funnel: the government, and the family. Pro-natal policies may not figure directly into most women's WiSK decisions, but they set the stage, teaching us that the family is deeply valued in our society. Our own families also provide a backdrop, giving us positive experiences we may one day hope to emulate for our own kids, or negative ones we hope to protect them from. Finally come the personal circumstances at the very bottom of the funnel: the factors at the fore of the decision making process. Our ability to find a suitable life partner, our educational goals, our career aspirations, our sense of independence—each of these personal factors impact WiSK decisions, and each ebbs and flows as we grow older. With so many factors swirling around in the funnel, it's no wonder that WiSK decisions are often made and changed several times in a woman's life.

CHAPTER THREE
The Contraceptive Revolution

In 1960, the WiSK game changed. That's when the Pill—an effective, safe oral contraceptive—was officially approved. As a result, women could have the exact number of children they wanted, when they wanted.[150] Family planning became more reliable than ever before.

Fast-forward sixty years to 2020: this so-called contraceptive revolution is still rocking the political boat. Abortion, sex education curricula, and the Pill itself continue to make news headlines. Just look at American president Donald Trump. He's filled his administration with anti-abortion and anti-birth control activists. That's led many women to worry that they'll suddenly lose access to the contraceptives they've relied on their entire adult lives.[151] Poland elicited its fair share of media attention in recent years. In the fall of 2016, a proposal to ban abortion was finally put to rest—but it took tens of thousands of protestors.[152] And there's plenty of drama right here at home. In Ontario, (mainly religious) parents have been protesting the introduction of a new sex education curriculum since 2015. Some have picketed at Queen's Park, while others kept their children home from classes.[153] Progressive Conservative leader Patrick Brown even campaigned for the leadership on the promise that he'd revoke the curriculum changes made by the Liberals.[154] So, to call it a "revolution" is not an overstatement; contraception has made waves all over the world for half a century.

What does this mean for women who are trying to plan (or prevent) a pregnancy? For starters, women should be empowered to choose the contraceptive method that's best for them—without worrying they'll be shamed, judged, or suddenly denied access to it. Second, to make these important choices, women—and men—need to know all their options. Formal sex education in school is a good starting point, but it isn't enough, as we'll see. Third and finally, awareness is useless without access. No matter their income, employment status, age, or geographic location, women need to be able to get the contraceptives they want. They also need power and confidence, so they can talk about using those contraceptives with their partners.

Though I provide some practical guidelines, this chapter is not a how-to manual. Nor is it intended to influence women's contraceptive choices. The last thing women need is more people telling them what to do with their own bodies. Rather, I aim to arm women with data—statistics, studies, and demographic trends—that they can use to make their own informed decisions.

Questions you'll get answers to:

▶ *Which contraceptives should you rely on to ensure you have the number of children you want, when you want?*

▶ *Why are some women more likely to use contraception than others?*

▶ *How can you ensure you (or your children) have reliable access to contraceptives?*

▶ *Abstinence is the most effective contraceptive—but is it realistic?*

▶ *How do women decide to keep or terminate unplanned pregnancies?*

▶ *In what circumstances is abortion a realistic option? What are its potential consequences?*

Putting Women in the Driver's Seat

If you look at only the numbers, it seems like the Pill was the spark that changed fertility trends. After its release—shocker!—unwanted pregnancies started dropping dramatically.[155]

But contraceptives don't fully explain WiSK trends. In the 1960s, women weren't only *having* fewer children; they started *wanting* fewer children. The Pill just gave these women a means to the ends they were after. It gave them control over their bodies, so they could mold their life course the way they wanted. If life is a highway (or even a public transit system), then contraception puts women in the driver's seat.

It especially helps women who want to Have It All. An unplanned pregnancy can disrupt—or destroy—a career.[156] There's nothing like maternity leave to bump you out of line for a promotion.

Despite its life-changing potential, it's taking us surprisingly long to hop on the contraception bandwagon. Though most North American women say they use some form of contraception, they admit they're far from consistent. So it's no surprise that roughly one third of pregnancies in Canada are still unplanned.[157]

Why is this happening when we have safe, simple tools that could prevent it? Some of the answer has to do with consistency and accuracy.

Let's start with the facts. Most contraceptives fall into one of five categories:

1. Intrauterine devices (IUDs), which prevent fertilization for years after they're inserted.

2. Barrier methods, like condoms, that physically keep sperm from reaching the egg.

3. Hormonal methods, such as the Pill, which prevent ovulation.

4. Sterilization—having your "tubes tied"—which makes women physically incapable of conceiving.

5. Natural methods, such as tracking and withdrawal.

Some of these methods are better than others. "Tier one" methods are best because they're foolproof: they depend least on proper use.[158] Tier two methods are only as good as the people using them, and most people aren't using them very well. Condoms, for example, are supposed to be 98 percent effective. Many (mistakenly) interpret this number to mean that, of every one hundred condom uses, two will result in pregnancy. Even better, the Pill is said to be 99.9 percent effective. So we think it's infallible, with a mere 0.1 percent of pill users getting pregnant.

But these rates refer to contraceptive "efficacy": how many pregnancies are prevented when the method is used perfectly.[159] Typical use, however, is far from perfect. Contraceptive "effectiveness" describes the number of pregnancies prevented by *typical* use.[160]

For example, many people who use condoms only use them sometimes. Others use expired condoms, or unknowingly use them with lubricants that reduce their efficacy. Women who rely on the Pill often say they take it several hours late, or forget altogether. These imperfect—yet typical—uses of contraceptives render them less effective than they would be, if used properly. Specifically, the Pill's effectiveness drops to roughly 90 percent with typical use.[161] And condoms are only 82 percent effective with typical use.

It seems like a no-brainer: given that they're virtually infallible, anyone trying to avoid pregnancy should opt for a tier one method like an IUD. Yet most North American women rely on tier two methods. The most popular contraceptive is condoms. Fifty-four percent of Canadians report them as their preferred method.[162] Another 44 percent say they use oral contraception, making it the second most widely used. At some point in their reproductive lives, over half of women use the Pill.[163] Shockingly, the third most popular method of "protection" is withdrawal, at 12 percent. (Note that these numbers don't add up to 100 percent because some people use two types of contraception at once. For example, some women who are on the Pill also use condoms.)

And many Canadians don't use any form of contraception at all. In 2011, Statistics Canada reported on sexually active 15-to-24-year-olds who said they were trying to avoid pregnancy: 15.5 percent admitted they didn't use contraception the last time they had sex.[164] But that rate varied by region: 28 percent of those in the territories were having unprotected sex, while 20 percent in B.C. and Ontario were.

The question is: why? Why would women who don't want kids use an unreliable method, or have unprotected sex? Often, outside factors keep them from getting or using contraceptives. Using, misusing, or forgoing contraception doesn't happen on a whim. Sociologists have long pointed to social factors that shape contraceptive behaviour. Here are a few of the most important ones:

1. Education

I mean two things here: the first is learning about sex and contraception. Many adults are mystified by it. In a study of over 4,100 women, roughly 45 percent thought the Pill and condoms were more effective than they actually are.[165] In another study of 1,800 sexually active men and women, one in four women and over half of the men admitted they knew little or nothing about contraception.[166] Forty percent said they didn't think birth control mattered at all.

Others are misinformed, and afraid of unproven side effects.[167] For example, many women are afraid to have IUDs inserted because they fear the outdated myth of IUD-induced infertility. Their doctors might make matters worse. One study showed that 30 percent of health care providers thought IUDs were unsafe for women who'd never given birth.[168] We now know that IUDs don't jeopardize women's ability to have children in the future. But because of this misinformation, many women are reluctant to try the most reliable form of birth control out there. Sex education can help, by arming women with the practical information they need from a young age.

The second thing I mean by education is schooling itself. One Canadian study looked at school attendance and accidental pregnancy rates.[169] It revealed that more schooling reduced the chances of becoming a teen mom by two to three percent. But these researchers also saw that regular attendance had little effect for women over the age of eighteen—those who'd graduated. So just being in school—physically showing up to class—can help prevent teen pregnancy.

And the more school you do, the better protected you are. Women who complete more formal education are more likely to use contraceptives. They also use them more effectively. In part, that's because they learn more about contraception and the proper ways to use it.

But it's also because of motivation. As I discussed in the last chapter, more highly educated women have a greater incentive to prevent untimely pregnancies. They have more to lose—namely, an education and well-paying career—so they're stricter about contraception. They may be more insistent on condom use, or take the Pill more consistently.

That said, even the smallest amount of education is better than nothing. One study looked at school policies put in place in Malawi, Uganda, and Ethiopia in the mid-1990s.[170] These policies did away with school enrolment fees, so girls were much more likely to attend and graduate. Those who completed just one additional year of schooling said they wanted smaller families. The extra schooling decreased desired family size by 34 percent in Malawi and Ethiopia, and by 11 percent in Uganda. And because they were learning about contraception, going to school also helped these women *have* the smaller number of children they wanted.

Lastly, higher education gives women confidence. They gain a sense of ownership over their bodies. More highly educated women believe they have *the right* to contraception. Those who opt for the Pill don't feel they need to consult their partners about it. And those who prefer condoms are better able to negotiate proper, consistent use with their partners.

As for men, higher education is also a plus. When both partners are more highly educated, they tend to be more egalitarian, make more decisions together, and communicate better about WiSK decisions. On the other hand, couples who are less educated communicate less and hold more traditional family ideals. This can lead them to have more children overall, and to start having them early.[171]

2. Income

Education and income are usually connected. So, the financial stability that tends to come along with higher education is related to contraceptive use. For example, women in the highest income quintile are twice as likely to use contraceptives than women in the lowest quintile (20.5 percent versus 10 percent).[172]

Part of the problem is affordability. Take IUDs as an example: they are very reliable, but they can also be expensive. In Ontario, some IUDs are free for women up to the age of 24 under OHIP+.[173] Women older than 24 could rely on providers like Planned Parenthood Toronto: they'll insert hormonal

IUDs for $380. But even that expense is impossible to cover if you're unemployed, or don't have benefits. In some places, inserting an IUD can cost up to $1,000 if you don't have health coverage through your employer.[174]

Other methods—like the Pill—aren't covered by Canada's free health care system either. As a result, between one quarter and one third of Canadian women have to pay for birth control.[175] Without employer-provided health care benefits, these women turn to more affordable—but less effective—methods, like condoms. So it's no surprise that unplanned pregnancies are more common among low-income earners.

American women are even more likely to say cost keeps them from using contraception. The Affordable Care Act reduced the cost of birth control for many. Yet that newfound affordability remains in political jeopardy. The cost of the Pill is especially problematic. After all, women must pay to visit a clinic to get their prescription, then pay each time they refill it. When the cost becomes too much, they switch to condoms.[176] Those especially desperate to cut costs stop using contraception altogether.

3. Race

Black and Latina women are less likely to use contraception.[177] Those who do use it typically rely on condoms, whereas white women are more likely to use the Pill.[178] So racialized women are more likely to get accidentally pregnant, and have abortions. This holds even after controlling for income. In other words, cost isn't what's keeping these women from preventing unwanted pregnancy.

So what *is*? Some racialized groups say they distrust certain types of contraception. That's because some family planning programs have a long history of discrimination. In the past, some racialized groups were sterilized as part of a eugenics agenda.[179] Remembering this history, some Black, Latina, and other racialized women are doubtful about birth control. They say they fear the government is trying to reduce their population by promoting birth control.

4. Convenience and Accessibility

Given the higher price of other methods, it makes sense that condoms are the most widely used contraceptive. They're also available everywhere. Many health clinics and university dormitories even hand them out for free. And they can be bought at the last minute, unlike tier-one contraceptives that require medical appointments, consultations, prescription pick-ups, or even surgeries.

Health coverage doesn't solve all of our problems, though. It can be hard to coordinate visits to the doctor and prescription refills.[180] Doctors are rarely available at convenient times for our work, school, and social schedules. When it comes to the Pill, there's also a limit on how many refills you can get at once. That means you have to make time to return to the pharmacy every few months. Studies show that these inconveniences make women use the Pill inconsistently. If it was available over-the-counter, women could purchase it without making a doctor's appointment, and outside of pharmacy hours. The problem is, health insurance might not cover the Pill if it's offered over-the-counter.

Accessibility poses a problem not only for low-income earners, but also for teenagers. Few teens feel comfortable discussing sex with their parents, let alone asking them for help choosing a contraceptive. That's why many go without protection altogether. Those who do use some form of contraception rely on easily accessible, affordable condoms. They'd be better off using tier one methods, but without their parents' health coverage—and consent—their options are limited.

In short, there are a lot of good options out there. But there are also a lot of barriers keeping women from using them. To be in the driver's seat and take control of their fertility, women need:

- to be fully informed about tier-one options. That means understanding that they're the most effective, and also that they're safe.
- these tier-one options to be free and convenient to get.

The biggest problem—and, as we'll see, the easiest one to fix—is knowledge. Of 4,144 women who got counseling about birth control, 71 percent chose an IUD or implant.[181] So when women are informed, they choose the tier-one method that offers them the best protection.

"Stealthing" and the Fight for Control

In January 2017, a man was convicted of rape.[182] After meeting on Tinder, the pair had agreed to have sex at her place. He eventually asked her if he could take his condom off—and though she refused, he did it anyway.

This act of "stealthing"—secretly removing a condom during sex—turns what may have started as consensual sex into non-consensual sex. Stealthing puts women at risk of pregnancy (and STIs), even though they've insisted on and think they *have* used protection. It's yet another way women who want to avoid pregnancy may find themselves unable to, despite the availability of contraceptives.

In a study that made news headlines, Alexandra Brodsky (2017), a legal fellow at the National Women's Law Centre, spoke with survivors of stealthing. The women Brodsky spoke with weren't just scared about pregnancy; they felt they had been violated. For example, when he told her he wanted to have sex without a condom, one of the women said: "'I'm really not OK with that, I'm currently not on birth control. My exact words were, 'that's not negotiable ... if that's a problem with you, that's fine. I'll leave.'" After he removed his condom anyway, the woman recalled: "it was such a blatant violation of what we'd agreed to. I set a boundary. I was very explicit." So, contraceptives are rightly praised for giving women power and control over their own bodies. But survivors of stealthing feel they have had that sense of empowerment taken away.

Stealthing is not the only practice that denies women control. In relationships that are abusive in other ways, fights over contraception are common. Consider "reproductive coercion": when men pressure their partners, verbally and/or physically, into having children.[183] Stealthing can be a form of reproductive coercion. So can withholding or throwing out birth control pills. Some men might explicitly insist that their partners get pregnant, using threats and violence to coerce them. Unfortunately, these tactics are often successful: studies show that women who have repeat abortions are often victims of reproductive control.[184]

Even when their partners don't want them to get pregnant, women in abusive relationships typically use less effective birth control methods than women in healthy relationships. Namely, women with abusive partners use condoms most often, though they're often inconsistent. With the threat of violence or abuse looming, it's harder for these women to insist their partners wear condoms. On the other hand, women in healthy relationships often use the Pill.[185]

What all of these scenarios have in common is a struggle for power and control. Stealthing, reproductive coercion, and a refusal to respect a woman's preferred method are all ways that men try to assert their power. These controlling tactics are most likely to arise when there are big differences between partners—for example, when a man is much older than his partner, has more education, or earns more money.[186] If a woman truly believes her partner is more powerful, she may be uncomfortable "demanding" things—like condom use—from him.

The Risk of Ambivalence

But just because a woman's in a healthy relationship doesn't mean she's using contraception. Being in a serious relationship can generate mixed feelings about pregnancy. They may not be in the "Start" phase of the WiSK process, but women with long-term partners may also not be as averse to pregnancy as when they were single. In other words, they wouldn't be wholly upset if they became pregnant, and may even see some benefits.

When couples are ambivalent about getting pregnant—they don't necessarily want to, but aren't entirely opposed—they are less likely to use contraception consistently. For instance, casually dating couples are more likely to use contraception than those who live together. In one study, 37 percent of daters said they'd used a condom the last time they'd had sex. Only 19 percent of cohabiters did. And while 57 percent of the daters said they were relying on a hormonal or other long-term contraceptive, only 40 percent of cohabiters were.[187]

Since cohabiters are more emotionally and materially committed to each other, they may feel indifferent about having a child together. They don't actively try to get pregnant, but they don't feel strongly committed to preventing it either.

With Great Power Comes Great Responsibility

Many women like being in the driver's seat. They welcome the control that contraceptives like the Pill give them over their own fertility. But others say they resent having the onus for safe sex placed on them.

Young women may be the most reluctant. One study[188] looked at teens' views on contraception. It revealed two outlooks, neither of which help prevent pregnancy. First, many of the young women who participated said their partners were dismissive about birth control; they didn't think it was "their job." Since women are the ones who can get pregnant, these men said they should take responsibility for preventing it.[189]

Second, some young women *do* take responsibility for contraception—and they are harshly judged for it. The same study found that many young women who carry condoms are labelled sluts.[190] Male respondents said if they went home with a woman from a bar or nightclub, and she had her own condoms, they would think she was overly experienced—as though she *knew* she'd be having sex. Other studies revealed similar attitudes. In one, for instance, respondents said they thought there was a stigma against women who carried condoms.[191]

Women may also develop a reputation if they show that they know how to properly use condoms, or if they insist that their partner wear them. A woman who is "overly familiar" with sex and birth control might be labelled "easy." And a woman who insists on condoms might be accused of having many partners. Because word travels fast in tightly-knit social circles—like high schools—many teenage girls would rather risk unprotected sex than risk harming their reputation.

Women who proactively plan safe sex may develop a bad reputation. But women are also told birth control is their problem, not something their male partners should worry about. Given this, it's surprising teen pregnancy rates aren't higher.

Plan B: The Morning-After Pill

In a perfect world, every woman who wanted to avoid pregnancy could. But the world isn't perfect: contraceptives often fail—or aren't used at all—leaving many women looking for a Plan B.

Enter the "morning-after pill." Formally known as "emergency contraception," the morning-after pill is one of the best options after having unprotected sex, if a condom slips or breaks, or if a woman misses her Pill.[192]

There are, however, still problems with Plan B. Cost is one of them. Plan B costs between $25 and $65 per dose.[193] And while Plan B is available on the shelves of most Canadian drug stores, it's kept behind the counter in Saskatchewan and requires a prescription to access in Quebec.[194] Where prescriptions are needed, women may not be able to get a doctor's appointment within the three days that Plan B is most effective.

There are also many myths and misconceptions about Plan B. In one study, 40 percent of participants thought emergency contraception was "an abortion pill."[195] Another 40 percent said they thought they could use it as their regular birth control, instead of only in emergencies. Twelve percent thought Plan B could cause infertility, while 44 percent thought they could only take it the day after having unprotected sex. Finally, 72 percent were unaware that men could purchase Plan B; they thought women alone were allowed to.

The myths surrounding Plan B make women less likely to use it. Studies show that pregnant women who didn't take Plan B often consider having an abortion.[196] In other words, they're willing to terminate a pregnancy once it's conceived, but were unable or unwilling to use emergency contraception to prevent that pregnancy. They were either unable to access Plan B, unsure how it worked, or scared off by rumours of its negative consequences.

Plan C: Abortion

The absolute last resort for some unintentionally pregnant women is to have an abortion. Technically, abortion can be considered a form of birth control: just like the Pill or a condom, an abortion prevents an unwanted birth. And just like the Pill or a condom, abortions are easier to access for some women than others.

People have been studying abortions, how women decide to get them, and their consequences for at least fifty years. One classic study is Nancy Howell Lee's *The Search for an Abortionist* (1969). The book investigates what it was like to try to get an abortion fifty years ago, before it was legal in the United States. It's informed mainly by the experiences of 114 women who had abortions in the late 1960s—even two who had to perform self-induced abortions.

Then as now, women—particularly poor women—were the chief victims of social policy that outlawed abortion. Women who could afford to pay for secret procedures performed by competent doctors would do so—for a hefty price. But poorer women could afford only dangerous "back-alley abortions." They risked infertility and even death, as well as their reputations. Those who couldn't afford even these sketchy procedures had to endure the shame of an unwanted pregnancy.

Even just a few decades ago, unmarried mothers were harshly judged. Compared with men, women were most likely to bear the shame and expenses of unwanted children. That made sex far riskier for women than men. Yet—then as now—it was often men who made and enforced laws about abortion and birth control.

Despite those laws, an estimated one million abortions were carried out each year in the United States in the late 1960s. Those who sought and got abortions were influenced by what they thought was "normal." Gossip about abortions—though intended to shame its targets—could make the procedure seem all the more common. Gossip could also spread information, letting more women know that abortions were available, and who could perform them.

Today, things have changed dramatically. That said, abortions—and the laws, accessibility issues, and stigma surrounding them—are certainly coloured by this history. In Canada, most abortions are performed as surgical procedures, so they happen in hospitals or clinics. While all hospitals have the surgical infrastructure needed to perform abortions, only a handful actually do. Abortion clinics are available to fill the gap, but they're mostly concentrated in cities. Women who live in the country are forced to take time off work and make long trips to clinics to get an abortion.[197]

It was not until 2017 that Prince Edward Island finally began providing abortion services within its borders. Before then, PEI residents had to travel out of province to receive an abortion. So we've made some great progress. But we can't forget that the PEI provincial government—like many others across Canada—still only covers the costs of abortions performed at hospitals, not private clinics.[198]

When abortions are expensive and time consuming, it discourages women from getting them. High costs and travel time are especially big turn-offs for women who earn low-incomes and may not be able to take time away from work. Unfortunately, these are the women who are at the greatest risk for unwanted pregnancies to begin with.[199] For example, how is a 15-year-old girl who lives in rural Manitoba with her single mother supposed to get downtown to an abortion clinic, let alone pay for the procedure?

Stigma is another barrier, just like it was for the women Howell Lee studied fifty years ago. A surprising number of doctors are against abortion for personal reasons. In one recent study, a woman reported her family physician had picketed abortion clinics.[200] On the other hand, many doctors aren't opposed to abortions in principle, but they are not trained or willing to perform them. Some see the threats, harassment, and even violence by pro-life protestors and think it's easier to stay out of it.

Pro-life attitudes pose yet another barrier. March for Life rallies continue to draw thousands in Canada.[201] Protestors station themselves outside of abortion clinics and harass everyone going in and out. Some groups have even attempted to outlaw or re-regulate abortion. Several private member bills have been introduced in the last decade aimed at passing legislation that would restrict women's abortion access. For instance, the 2012 March for Life rally on Parliament Hill was meant to help pass these types of laws. These Marches continue today.

But as Stephen Harper said in a 2011 CBC documentary, "if you want to diminish the number of abortions, you've got to change hearts and not laws." Many anti-abortion advocates have followed Harper's advice. They use scare and intimidation tactics—rather than laws—to dissuade women from having abortions.[202] These advocates make their views known through blogs, PSAs, and advertising campaigns. There, they represent women as helpless victims of abortion, taken advantage of by doctors who failed to explain their options. Or they vilify them as selfish, immoral women who refuse to let a child "interrupt" their social lives.

In sum, we know that many women seek abortions, but not all who want them can get them. To help women time their pregnancies the way they want, we need to remove those barriers. That means we need more hospitals and clinics offering abortions; publicly funded procedures; more doctors who are trained to provide abortions; and protection from pro-choice protestors for those doctors.[203] And, as I'll discuss below, we need to do a better job of being available to, and non-judgmental towards, our daughters. They need to feel comfortable asking us for help when they need it.

Breaking Down Barriers

Despite the many roadblocks in their way, many women still seek abortions. One in three Canadian women will have an abortion in their lifetime.[204] Almost 98,000 abortions were reported in Canada in 2016. The majority of abortions—over 21,000—were reported among women between the ages of 20 and 24. And this may be a low estimate: because abortion is stigmatized, many women may not admit that they've had one. So it's possible these numbers don't reflect the true extent of abortion in Canada.[205]

The tables on page 72 show large numbers of abortions, which suggest two things. First, no matter the barriers, some unexpectedly pregnant women see abortion as their best option. They will sacrifice time, money, and reputation to get one. Second, high abortion rates suggest we're failing to meet Ca-

Table 1
Induced Abortions in Canada (2016)

Province or territory	Abortions reported by hospitals	Abortions reported by clinics	Total number of abortions
Newfoundland and Labrador	138	840	978
Prince Edward Island	0	0	0
Nova Scotia	1,908	0	1,908
New Brunswick	827	0	827
Quebec	7,881	15,512	23,393
Ontario	9,907	28,476	38,383
Manitoba	2,130	1,538	3,668
Saskatchewan	1,878	204	2,082
Alberta	1,719	11,229	12,948
British Columbia	3,950	9,166	13,116
Yukon	116	0	116
Northwest Territories	277	0	277
Nunavut	68	0	68
Total reported	**30,799**	**66,965**	**97,764**

Source: Based on data from Canadian Institute for Health Information (https://www.cihi.ca/en/induced-abortions-reported-in-canada-in-2016).

Table 2
Method of Abortions Reported by Canadian Hospitals (excluding Quebec) in 2014

Method of abortion	Number of induced abortions reported by hospitals	Percentage of induced abortions reported by hospitals
Surgical procedures only	21,903	88.5%
Surgical and medical procedures	1,457	5.9%
Medical procedures only	1,269	5.1%
Other	110	0.4%
Total	**24,739**	**100.0%**

Source: Canadian Institute for Health Information (https://www.cihi.ca/sites/default/files/.../induced_abortion_can_2014_en_web.xlsx).

nadian women's contraceptive needs. Often, women who seek abortions say they were misusing or afraid of using contraception. Over 20 percent say they didn't use any form of contraception at all.[206] More accessible contraceptives—and the female empowerment needed to negotiate their use—would help more women keep their WiSK plans on track.

Some women are more likely to fall in this second group than others. One study found immigrant women seeking abortions were less likely to have been using hormonal contraception when they conceived.[207] Fully 62.6 percent of these women said they didn't think the Pill was healthy, while 57.4 percent said they were afraid to use an IUD and 24.8 percent said they had trouble getting any kind of birth control at all. Most often, they said they didn't have enough money to afford it. Happily, these attitudes and behaviours change over time, with women who live in Canada for over five years adopting more positive attitudes towards contraceptives and beginning to use them.

When is Abortion the Best Option?

Pro-life advocates say abortions are always bad.[208] In the past, they would argue for the "rights" of fetuses. But today, they position themselves as feminists who just want what's best for women.

Take the Silent No More campaign as an example. Its creators say it raises awareness around the "devastation abortion brings to women and men" (2018). The Silent No More website features testimonials from women who had abortions, and men who "regret" their "lost fatherhood." Those who don't want to publicize their experiences are asked to "register their regret," adding their names to the list of 5,361 women and 625 men who have anonymously declared they regret their decision to have an abortion.[209]

Pro-choice advocates argue the other side of the debate. A good example of a pro-choice campaign is 1 in 3. It's named after the statistic that one in three women will have an abortion in their lifetime. Like Silent No More, the 1 in 3 website also shares testimonials, except these ones are from women who are thankful they got to choose for themselves. By sharing these stories, the campaign hopes to "end the stigma and shame women are made to feel about abortion" and "build a culture of compassion, empathy, and support for access to basic health care."

Looked at side by side, these two campaigns show that no two experiences with abortion are the same. Some women regret their decision to have an abortion. But others attribute their success and happiness to getting one. Ultimately, the decision to continue or abort a pregnancy is an entirely personal one. But many women thinking about abortion still lack the facts. What are the risks? How have other women made this decision? How do they typically react, once it's over? If you decide to have an abortion, are you likely to regret it?

Social science has provided decades worth of data—and the testimonies of countless women—that can answer these questions. First, there are medical risks that come along with abortions. Some of these are the same risks that all surgical or medical procedures carry. But in addition, abortion can have emotional or psychological costs. Some women say they experience sadness, stress, or shame.[210] Doctors acknowledge that these are entirely normal reactions.[211] But for most women, these feelings go away after days or weeks. And for most women, feelings of stress are reduced—not increased—by aborting an unwanted pregnancy.

As for the decision-making process, pro-life campaigns tell us that women agonize over whether or not they should have an abortion. It's painted as a painful, even traumatizing, decision that women remember—and regret—their entire lives.[212] This belief is reflected in laws in several US states that can force women to receive counselling, undergo a waiting period, or view an ultrasound of the fetus before they are allowed to abort it.

Such laws imply that choosing an abortion is somehow different from choosing any other type of medical surgery—so different that it requires special intervention and guidance from practitioners. But in reality, many women are confident in their decision right from the start. They make an appointment with their doctor feeling certain that they will receive an abortion. And more often than not, they follow through with confidence. For instance, one study found that 90 percent of women felt sure about what to choose.[213] These women were equally or more assured of their decision than women who made other healthcare decisions. Specifically, they felt more confident about getting an abortion than other women did about having a mastectomy after being diagnosed with breast cancer; about receiving prenatal testing after being infertile; or about using antidepressants while pregnant.[214] So, pro-life advocates make the decision to have an abortion seem harder than it actually is. Many other healthcare decisions are, in fact, more difficult and stressful for women to make.

On the other hand, some women are less confident in their decision. But when we look at their beliefs and values, it's obvious why. Women who are less assured about their choice tend to endorse pro-life myths about abortions. For example, they are likely to think that "abortion causes breast cancer," or that "childbirth is safer than abortion." Interestingly, these women have abortions anyway, despite their fears. That they follow through in the face of these (mistaken) beliefs shows their determination not to continue their pregnancy.

How can these women be so sure that abortion is the "right thing"? In many cases, they're confident because they knew they weren't ready to become parents. They feel they're making the best choice not only for themselves, but also for the fetus. If they're single, earning a low income, or in unstable relationships, women may opt for an abortion because they believe they aren't able to give a child a good life.[215] Others are already parents. They know they can't have another child without compromising the care they give to their other kids.

When it comes to reactions, post-abortion regret is rare. Ninety-five percent of women in one study[216] said they did not regret having abortions. They did react emotionally, but that's normal and understandable. Those reactions also subside with time. On the whole, the majority of women say they have better self-esteem and are more satisfied with life after getting an abortion. They are also less stressed, depressed, and anxious.

These positive results are most common for women who

get support from their friends and family. They can talk openly and without judgment about their abortions, so they feel supported and confident in their decision.[217] On the other hand, women who think their friends and family will disapprove don't talk about their abortions.[218] As a result, they tend to feel unsupported, guilty, and ashamed.

In short, few women find abortion to be the life-ruining trauma that pro-life advocates say it is. Those who struggle are often not upset by the abortion itself. Rather, they're *made* to feel guilty by pro-life attitudes.

Overall, abortions aren't problems in and of themselves. The problem is that too many women who are trying to avoid pregnancy must resort to this "Plan C." Whether it's because of a lack of education, an abusive partner, an inability to pay for contraception, or any of the other barriers discussed in this chapter, these women have found themselves pregnant when they don't want to be. We have to make abortions available to the women who want and are unable to access them. But equally important, we also have to develop better contraceptive solutions that prevent unplanned pregnancies altogether.

Genetic Testing and Termination

Some women who have abortions want to have a child; they just don't want the fetus they are carrying.

Thanks to recent medical advances, women can know things about their children before they're even born. Many expecting parents are excited to learn the sex of their baby from an ultrasound. But others are looking for information about their fetus's development. For women who conceive in their late thirties or forties, fears of irregularities abound. Some of these women opt for amniocentesis tests, which screen their fetuses for such irregularities. When they learn their child is not developing normally, they may choose to terminate the pregnancy.

Usually, they make that choice based on the irregularity's severity. For example, they might abort if they are told their child will be born in great pain and will only live for a few days. When parents expect their child will be born with such a severe, debilitating condition, up to 85 percent terminate the pregnancy.[219]

Amniocentesis tests are known to carry risks, including miscarriage. That deters some women from taking them. But as testing procedures become less invasive and more reliable, more and more expectant parents use them. For example, a DNA-based test called MaterniT21 screens for Down syndrome. All it takes is a blood sample from the mother.[220] When these tests reveal Down syndrome, parents abort the pregnancy between 60 and 90 percent of the time.

Some research suggests this happens less often today. As our society becomes more accepting of people with disabilities, fewer parents feel the need to screen for or abort fetuses that are developing irregularly. But other studies suggest expectant parents don't receive enough guidance when making the decision to abort or keep a fetus. Many doctors and even genetic counselors report feeling inadequately trained to provide parents with the support they need when they learn that their pregnancy is not "normal." And many parents still feel pressured to abort a fetus that will be "abnormal" in any way. Though we're making progress, people with disabilities are still stigmatized. There's also plenty of social pressure to have "normal" children.[221]

For many, this decision is riddled with a fear of the unknown. Most likely, these expectant parents don't know what the life of a child with a disability would look like. So, they try to recall their experiences with people with disabilities: what they've seen or heard in the past. Some actively seek out parents with children who have disabilities. By talking with them, they try to imagine what their own lives would be like, should they choose to have their own child with a disability.[222] Those who can get comfortable with these adjusted expectations will continue their pregnancy.

The Abstinence Myth

In the 2004 cult classic *Mean Girls*, Coach Carr gives his students a bizarre lecture. He perfectly captures the awkward embarrassment of every high school teacher who's been forced to teach sex education as he yells: "Don't have sex, because you *will* get pregnant … and die! Don't have sex in the missionary position, don't have sex standing up, just … don't do it. OK? Promise?" But even he recognizes the futility of asking a classroom of 17-year-olds to abstain. He ends his useless lecture holding out a box of condoms in defeat: "OK, now everybody take some rubbers."

Though many parents love the idea, abstinence doesn't work.[223] True, it's the only 100 percent effective method of birth control. But it's almost impossible for teens to adhere to.

Look at studies of "virginity pledges" as an example. Teens who vow to stay virgins until they get married are just as likely to have premarital sex as teens who don't take the pledge. But pledgers are less likely to use contraception.[224] They've never learned about any of the options available to them, so it's no surprise they don't use any. On the other hand, students who learn about a range of birth control options—including, but not limited to, abstinence—are much less likely to have unprotected sex or get pregnant.[225] In short, only teaching abstinence is just as bad as not teaching youth about sex at all.

In fact, teaching abstinence in schools might be driving teen pregnancy rates up. One American study showed that the more policies and state laws stress abstinence, the higher the average teen pregnancy and birth rates are.[226] The lowest rates of teen pregnancy are found in states where teens are taught about contraception.

Canada has teen pregnancy problems too, but they aren't as common. The pregnancy rate among Canadian teens has been declining over the past 25 years.[227] As the table on the next page shows, fewer Canadian teens give birth year after year—but there are still several thousand annually.

Though we're making progress, we can do better. For many, teen pregnancy has negative results, regardless of how much the mother loves her child. Teen mothers are less likely to receive prenatal care, for example, and both they and their children are at risk for poor mental and physical health. Teen parents are also less likely to complete high school, as are their children.[228] And teen moms and their families are also more

Table 3
Live Births by Age of Mother in Canada

Age of mother	2009	2010	2011	2012	2013
All ages	380,863	377,213	377,636	381,869	380,323
Under 15 years	104	102	99	79	78
15 to 19 years	15,534	14,554	13,436	12,843	11,645
20 to 24 years	57,778	55,217	53,478	52,170	50,309
25 to 29 years	116,878	114,069	113,628	114,045	111,495
30 to 34 years	120,734	121,613	124,349	127,914	130,744
35 to 39 years	57,733	58,905	59,656	61,427	62,567
40 to 44 years	11,364	11,881	12,207	12,671	12,710
45 to 49 years	605	577	708	695	734
Age not stated	133	295	75	25	41

Source: Statistics Canada (2017), Live Births by Age of Mother, Canada, Provinces and Territories (http://www5.statcan.gc.ca/cansim/a26?lang=eng&id=1024503&p2=46).

likely to live in poverty.[229] For these reasons, many parents try to keep their teenage daughters childfree, and many teenage girls try to avoid pregnancy.

There are two ways we can help. The first is formal sex education.[230] Youth who are required to learn a structured sex education curriculum are more likely to start having sex at older ages. They're also less likely to have unprotected sex.[231] And, thanks to their more consistent use of contraceptives, they tend to have kids later, at older ages.[232]

Despite these facts, some Canadians vehemently oppose sex education. Here are some of the myths they like to spread—and the research disproving them:

▶ Myth: *Families—not schools—should educate their children about sex.*[233]

▶ Fact: *Many parents don't have complete, reliable information about sexuality and contraception. And many parents aren't comfortable talking about sex with their children. Teaching sex education in schools ensures every student gets the information they need.*

▶ Myth: *Sex education encourages youth to have sex.*[234]
Fact: *47 percent of youth who get sex education wait longer to have sex.*[235] *And 63 percent of sex education programs improve students' use of contraceptives.*

- ▶ Myth: *Children shouldn't be exposed to the adult concept of sex.*[236]
- ▶ Fact: *Teens aren't as naïve as their parents like to believe. Many teens will have sex before graduating from high school.*

For these reasons, we need to give young people the information they need to make informed choices. If girls know about safe sex and contraception, they'll be better equipped to make smart decisions when they eventually start having sex.

A second way to reduce teen pregnancies is by making birth control more accessible. Doctors in most provinces of Canada are bound by confidentiality clauses for patients 16 years of age and over, but many teens don't know that. They fear their parents will find out if they ask their doctor for the Pill or an IUD. Rather than risk getting into trouble, many youth decide to go without protection.

In sum, denying youth knowledge of and access to contraceptives doesn't keep them from having sex; they just end up having unprotected sex. If we want to help our daughters have bright futures, we should:

- champion sexual education,
- object to programs that push abstinence, and
- ensure our children have access to contraceptives.

Final Thoughts

Women have much more control over their futures than they did 60 years ago, before birth control was introduced. But as we've seen, we still have a long way to go before all women can take advantage of contraception.

Women who have carefully planned when they want to have children—or who want to avoid having children indefinitely—can guarantee their plans succeed by choosing a tier one method of birth control, like an IUD. But there are steps we need to take before all women can make this choice:

- Women need to be informed: taught their options, and taught that they are safe.
- Birth control needs to be made accessible: affordable and easy to get.

- We must work to end stigma and shame. Young women need to be able to access birth control without worrying what their parents will think. And women of all ages should feel empowered to choose for themselves, without worrying what their partners might think or do.

Contraception is one of the keys to helping women actualize their WiSK plans. It's time they were empowered to use it.

CHAPTER FOUR
Baby Mania:
The Power of Popular Beliefs

You are probably familiar with Roy Lichtenstein's famous 1960s pop-art piece—an enlarged and stylized comic-strip panel depicting a sobbing young woman declaring "I can't believe I forgot to have a baby!" The image—which today is almost ubiquitous, available not only as a poster but on coffee mugs and T-shirts sold on Amazon and Etsy—is as relevant now as it was during the post-war baby boom. As you know from the last chapter, that's when the Pill was getting popular. Yet many women were warned not to use it. They were told they should *want* to succumb to their maternal instincts—not stifle them. Today, women are still being cautioned about the dangers of delaying motherhood. They're told that, when it's too late and they're no longer able to conceive, they'll regret their WiSK decisions. As Lichtenstein put it, women are so busy living their lives, they "forget" to have kids—only to regret it later.

These popular beliefs are the focus of this chapter. Here, I record the many stereotypes, debates, and understandings of "right and wrong" that shape our views of parenthood. These beliefs underpin what French writer Corinne Maier describes as "baby mania." In her book, *No Kids: Forty Reasons Not to Have Children*, Maier says our society is obsessed with babies. She points out how we glorify motherhood, making it seem like the most rewarding experience life can offer. It's easy to see what she means. The films we watch, the living arrangements we choose, the conversations we have with our friends and family—so much of our lives revolve around finding a partner and starting a family.

This baby mania has been around forever. Decades ago, our beliefs about marriage and childbearing were stronger. People felt more obligated to conform to them. But a look at the different families in your neighbourhood shows how much things are changing. We're still obsessed with babies, but today, we're more relaxed about what counts as a family. For example, look at couples who have kids without getting married. People have children out of wedlock because they want children, not a wedding.[237] Just a few decades ago, that would have been scandalous. There are lots of other good examples:

- Some 2SLGBTQ+ couples get married and have children.
- Some women choose to have children by themselves.
- Some people start families much later in life.
- Some choose to never have kids at all.

That said, many people still hold strong beliefs about The Family. And many people are pressured to conform to those beliefs. In this chapter, I look at their effects. How do these beliefs shape WiSK plans? Where do they fit into the factor funnel? And what happens when women decide—or are forced— to go against these beliefs?

As we will see, beliefs are incredibly powerful. At some level, we all have a desire to belong: to fit in and be part of the group. Doing parenthood—dreaming about it, debating whether you want it, delaying it, and eventually making it happen—makes us members of the biggest club that's ever existed. In our baby-obsessed culture, it's a club you grow up believing you'll be part of some day. So, beliefs *are* the factor funnel: they're what shape all the other factors. Without beliefs, there's no structure to swirl the other factors around into WiSK decisions.

Questions you'll get answers to:

▶ *What do people think it takes to be a good mother? What do they see as bad mothering?*

▶ *How old is "too old" to have your first child?*

▶ *How do these beliefs impact women's WiSK decisions? How do they play into feelings of shame, fear, and guilt?*

▶ *Do people's expectations of parenthood match up with their experiences?*

Good and Bad Moms

Comedian (and father) Louis C.K. has hilariously explained why parents don't judge other parents. "You know when you see a mother in McDonalds … or in a toy store, and she's melting down on her kid? She's like, 'Shut up. I hate you. You're ugly!' And people are standing around going, 'Oh my goodness, she's a horrible mother!' Well guess what? Those people aren't fucking parents! They don't have children. Because any *parents* who are in that store are thinking, 'What did that shitty kid do to that poor woman? That poor woman, I wish I could help.…'"

Public temper tantrums certainly attract a lot of attention. There's staring, whispering, and maybe even some unsolicited parenting advice. These looks and comments seem innocent, but they remind women that they're failing to live up to expectations.[238] Added up, these humiliating moments can make women feel like Bad Moms.

And it usually is women who get the brunt of it. In one study, Garner (2015) looked at family visits to the museum. She saw that staff and other museum visitors scrutinized mothers. Often, they found something to criticize about their parenting. But when it came to fathers, staff and visitors sympathized with them. Some were even praised for putting in such great effort.

Most of us agree about what makes a Good Mom.[239] Good Moms put their children first—their needs above all else.[240] They're on duty 24/7, to do whatever their children need.[241] Good Moms love their children unconditionally, and accept them for who they are. Their kids get the perfect balance of support and independence. Finally, Good Moms are patient, calm, attentive, and selfless.[242] To put their children's needs first, they control their own needs. They hide their stress, anger, and exhaustion so they don't upset their children.

These expectations are almost impossible to meet. Many women quickly realize how high these standards are after giving birth. In one study, women described the first few weeks of motherhood as "nightmarish"—like "a period of mourning for your old life".[243] Good Mothering did not come naturally, like they expected.

A period of adjustment is normal. But many women feel guilty when their "maternal instincts" don't kick in.[244] We make women believe that mothering should come naturally. There's a myth that genetic hardwiring makes women ideal caregivers. They automatically know how to care for their children, and feel immediate, unconditional love for them. We also make women believe that mothering should be pure bliss.[245] New motherhood is supposed to be the happiest time of your life.[246]

In reality, maternal instincts are largely a myth. Now, we *are* hardwired to defend our offspring, so we can survive as a species. But that's our survival instinct: an urge to protect our children from physical danger. It doesn't mean all women instinctively know how to be Good Moms. It's never easy to give another human unwavering patience and affection—never mind when you're exhausted, stressed, and even depressed. Like any other new responsibility, parents need time to figure out what they're doing. That learning phase is only made more stressful when we tell new mothers that they're lacking some maternal instinct.

The Baby Blues: How Sad Moms Became Bad Moms

Stress, mood swings, sadness, and irritability are common among new moms. *Most* mothers sing the baby blues for a week or two after giving birth. Although more serious and long-term, postpartum depression (PPD) is more common than many people realize. Up to one in five new mothers experience PPD.[247] It can also affect women who adopt, and partners who do not physically deliver their babies. We make things worse by believing that new mothers should be naturally overcome with joy. That makes struggling moms feel ashamed or abnormal.[248]

People have been researching PPD since at least the 1950s. Back then, it was seen as a sign that a woman was failing to adjust to her new motherly responsibilities.[249] Essentially, these "sad" moms were deemed Bad Moms. In the 1960s, doctors prescribed tranquilizers and anti-depressants to these women. The baby blues were seen as a temporary psychiatric problem that women could fix by taking their meds. In the '70s, feminists joined the chorus. They proposed new moms felt depressed because they were expected to stay home with their children. Without careers or goals outside of their family, feminists believed women lacked purpose. But, as more women started balancing work and family, many felt even *more* stressed.

Some anti-feminist backlash followed in the '80s. Then, working mothers were made out to be selfish Bad Moms. People accused them of prioritizing their careers over their kids. At this point, postpartum depression was no longer seen as a temporary issue. People viewed it as an abnormal illness requiring medical intervention. Things were only made worse by the growing belief that happy moms make for happy children. Feelings of sadness or stress were thought to negatively impact children's development. So, from the moment they conceived, women were pressured to express only positive emotions.

Today, we do a much better job of acknowledging the struggle new parents face. That said, PPD still isn't talked about as much as it should be. And when we do broach the subject, we still focus on changing the feelings of individual people. Rarely do we question the Good Mom ideal that leaves so many women feeling bad about themselves.[250]

Much more often, though, we do our best to forget about PPD. The feelings of hopelessness and guilt that come along with the condition aren't "supposed" to be part of new-parent bliss. Unlike selfless Good Moms who easily fall in love with their babies, women who experience PPD may feel overwhelmed and even resent their babies. These reactions go against our beliefs. They challenge the happy picture of new parenthood we've been taught to believe. That's why people point fingers at women who struggle with PPD. They're seen as strange and even crazy for "failing" to recognize the joys of motherhood. Some are reviled as Bad Moms. After all, they haven't set their own emotions aside to give their babies top priority.[251] So, we have come a long way, but we still assume that motherhood and negative emotions are incompatible.[252]

Of course, there are other causes of PPD too. Genes, life experiences, and especially sleep deprivation can be risk factors. But our beliefs about parenthood play an obvious role.[253] Amid baby mania, people become convinced they need to have the perfect pregnancy, birth, and baby. The pressure to be the perfect parent is overwhelming.

Even if PPD was 100 percent genetically determined, beliefs about parenthood would only make it worse. Those who struggle with PPD often feel guilty, ashamed, or unworthy of raising children. Impossibly high standards for being a Good Mom compound these feelings. Our beliefs just make parents feel even more inadequate.

Those beliefs also make it harder for people with PPD to get the support they need. Women who do come forward often say they're ashamed.[254] Instead of getting help, many women hide their PPD so they can avoid being called Bad Moms.

C-Sections and the Search for Selflessness

Just a few short weeks after meeting on reality TV show *Bachelor in Paradise*, now-celebrity couple Jade and Tanner Tolbert married. Two years later, they were expecting their first child. As social media influencers, the couple's journey to parenthood was splashed all over Instagram. Tanner even Instagrammed a photo of Jade in the midst of a clearly painful delivery. "Watching you give birth to our daughter was truly one of the most amazing things I have ever seen and I am so proud of you," read the caption. "I thought I loved you before … but the amount of respect and love I have for you now is even higher. I am so excited to watch you be a mom to our little girl. Oh, and you are kind of a badass for giving birth without pain meds or drugs."

According to Tanner, Jade was a Good Mom even before their daughter, Emerson, was born. Her drug-free delivery was only one of many sacrifices Jade made for her daughter. Her Instagram is essentially just a list of all the special measures she took while she and Tanner were trying to conceive, and throughout her pregnancy.

For most of their lives, women are taught to think of their bodies as baby-making vessels.[255] Before they've even hit puberty, girls are told to take care of themselves so they can have healthy babies someday. (Think of the parents who caution their daughters from sitting on cold surfaces that could damage their reproductive organs.) It's true that healthy women have better chances of having healthy babies. But this thinking implies that a woman's greatest purpose in life is to have children.

If something goes wrong during their pregnancy, women become Bad Moms for failing to prevent it. They're blamed for messing up their prenatal vitamins, or caving to their cravings, or stressing out, or exercising too hard or not hard enough. By contrast, fathers' contributions are rarely questioned. Birth defects and such are almost always assumed to happen because the mother failed to take care of her body.

As Tanner's Instagram shows, the act of childbirth itself also makes women Good or Bad Moms. Good Moms are supposed to be selfless, sacrificing their own needs to focus on their child's. Jade's drug-free, "natural" delivery fits the bill. Vaginal deliveries are seen as a rite of passage into womanhood.[256] The pain is an indoctrination into the selflessness of motherhood. Women who deliver vaginally, without drugs, sacrifice their bodies in a way that will permanently change them. They physically prove they aren't selfish, lazy, or any of the other things Bad Moms are accused of being.

On the other hand, caesarean sections ("C-sections" for short) are sometimes seen as taking the easy way out. That's especially the case if they're scheduled in advance or aren't medically necessary. Yet, some women have them anyway. They fear what childbirth will do to their bodies or to their sex lives. Some say they don't think their husbands will want them anymore after they give birth vaginally. They fear it will drive their partners into the arms of other women who haven't been "ruined" by childbirth.

In one study, a mother said her husband was relieved after she had an unplanned C-section. He said he'd worried what sex would be like after a vaginal delivery. His concerns ultimately drove this mother to have a planned C-section for their second child.[257]

They might hold their husbands' interest, but women who have planned C-sections risk being labeled Bad Moms. They've tried to preserve their bodies and their sex appeal. That makes some people see these women as selfish. They can't be Good

Moms because Good Moms are selfless, willing to sacrifice their bodies and relationships for their children. We tell women that for Good Moms, life is no longer about them. It's all about their child, and their husband should accept that.

The C-section stigma is hard to avoid, even when it's medically necessary. C-sections can make women feel disempowered. In the same study, another woman spoke about complications with her second pregnancy that forced her to have a C-section. Unable to give birth naturally, as she had for her first child, this woman said she felt like "a turkey on a platter." Doctors were carving into her body, taking away her sense of control. They were performing the act that *makes* women mothers—the selfless painful delivery—on her behalf.[258] It's as though a woman becomes less of a mother if she loses control over her delivery. If doctors intervene, she's stripped of that first opportunity to show her selfless commitment to her child.

Some mothers realize that selflessness is impossible—and undesirable. As burnout and PPD gain attention, so too does self-care. Some women even include self-care in their definition of Good Mothering.[259] In one study, a mother said she'd resent her child if she devoted all of her time and energy to them. Instead, she saw Good Mothering as taking time for herself so she'd have more energy for her child.

Without self-care, many new moms feel consumed by parenting. Since Good Moms are ultra-attentive, motherhood becomes their identity. It's a slippery slope, considering that everything changes once you give birth—even your name. Suddenly, you're "Mom," always referred to in terms of your new responsibilities. Even your partner starts calling you by your new name (and they also take on a new identity as "Dad" or "Mom"). Because it takes over their lives, motherhood is seen as the ultimate role women can aspire to fill.[260] Many see motherhood as a central part of female identity. It gives them purpose and fills their life with meaning.[261] So, Good Moms are often also thought to be "good women": those who have successfully achieved what's expected of them.

But not all women *want* to be defined by motherhood. Our beliefs about what makes a Good Mom are so strong that most women try to meet them. They try to be constantly attentive, but that means they start sacrificing other things, like their work, friendships, and relationships. Mothering becomes the all-consuming job our society tells women it should be—but it doesn't feel healthy or fulfilling. That's why so many women celebrate when they get to go back to work, or do something besides mother. Working, volunteering, and other pursuits give them a sense of purpose unrelated to their kids. And that gives them an identity free from the stress of Good Mothering and the shame of Bad Mothering.

That's not to say our belief in the Good Mom is wavering. The supermom trend is still going strong, which shows how little our beliefs have changed over the last several decades. Women are well aware of these impossibly high expectations. The fear of having to sacrifice their own needs to meet their children's makes plenty of women nervous to become moms. Those who value their careers, their relationships, and their own personal well-being fear they won't live up to Good Mom standards. But these expectations are bad for both mothers and children. Mothers who prioritize their children's needs over their own risk burnout. That means their children end up with poorer quality care in the end.

Child Freedom

No one pokes fun at the Good Mom better than Maier. Her bestselling book *No Kids*, which I mentioned earlier, was among the first in a series of famous admissions from mothers who regret having kids. Maier mixes humour—"Don't become a travelling feeding bottle"—with some dark personal admissions: "you will inevitably be disappointed with your child … we dream about wonderful children, but there are no wonderful children. They are people like me and you, and they fail, they do things you don't expect, they dream of things you don't even imagine, things that are pointless for you but not for them. So of course they have to disappoint you."[262] Just a few pages will make you question the baby mania that drives our lives.

A few years later, in 2013, Isabella Dutton was featured in the *Daily Mail* as "The mother who says having these two children is the biggest regret of her life." And in 2016, German novelist Sarah Fischer wrote *The Mother Bliss Lie: Regretting Motherhood*. Fischer says motherhood is actually miserable—not the best time of your life.

Many more women have voiced their regrets anonymously. The Facebook page "I Regret Having Children" features hundreds of posts like this one:

> My kids are 5 and 2 and I absolutely hate having them. The thought of having to wake up in the morning makes me want to scream every night. They make me miserable. I wish they didn't exist. I think I still love them but I'm not sure any more. They just annoy me all day. I try to get things done but I can never go longer than 10 minutes before 1 of them is screaming about something. My husband doesn't help with them much so I'm taking care of them all day. Every day. Non stop. I thought I wanted kids but now I know I don't. There are things you don't know if you will like them unless you try them. But sadly this is not one I can take back. I dream every day that I could live alone and in peace. I know that I am not a bad person for thinking this because I have [the] right to have feelings and opinions. I want to hear from you out there who feel the same. Tell me your story. So I know I'm not alone.

It's no wonder these women want to stay anonymous. Motherhood is painted as the most fulfilling thing they'll ever get to enjoy.[263] Women are supposed to cherish their children. They're told the sleepless nights and never-ending days of diaper changing are labours of love, outweighed by the joys of mothering. Up against these high expectations, women are reluctant to say they're disappointed with motherhood. It doesn't help that those who *have* spoken out are met with vicious backlash. Dutton, for example, was called "an utterly miserable, cold-hearted and selfish woman." These confessions come from a generation of women who often felt pressure to become parents. That used to be a guaranteed step in the life course—as unavoidable as getting a job. Amidst all the baby mania, it's no wonder they hopped on the bandwagon. They knew they'd face serious social repercussions if they didn't.

But today, more women are choosing not to have kids.[264] They see how overwhelming motherhood can be, and some want nothing to do with it. They opt to stay "free" from children.

It's a small fraction of women, though. Beliefs don't change overnight. Most people still think that everyone *should* have children, at some point.[265] At best, people who stay child free are confronted with shock almost every time a stranger learns of their decision. They're bombarded with questions about why they would willingly avoid parenthood. At worse, they're harshly judged—told they're selfish or unwomanly.

These negative reactions show we still hold traditional beliefs about The Family. That's no surprise; these beliefs go back hundreds of years. And those long-standing beliefs are hard to go up against. So, the small group of women who choose to stay child free face a lot of stigma—so much that many change their minds and have children after all.[266]

Just a few decades ago, having children was seen as the whole point of marriage.[267] It was unheard of for a woman to have a professional career. Likewise, stay-at-home dads didn't exist. People believed it was women's duty to raise the next generation, and men's duty to support their families financially.

All of these beliefs still persist even today. They make child freedom look bad to many. Childfree women are often called selfish, immature, and lazy. They're accused of shirking their responsibility for raising the next generation.[268] Some even think that childfree women must be "crazy" or emotionally unstable. As discussed, Good Moms and Good Women often mean the same thing.[269] So, women who stay childfree are often judged as bad people for refusing to live up to society's expectations.

A recent study captures how quick we are to judge.[270] People were asked to share their views on different groups of women: mothers, involuntarily childless women, and voluntarily childfree women.[271] Participants said mothers had the "warmest" personalities. They were admired. Involuntarily childless women got some pity. People assumed they *wanted* children, so they felt sympathetic. But childfree women got the worst of it. People said these women "disgusted" them. So, people see women favourably when they meet our expectations. Mothers uphold our beliefs, so they're admired. Women who stay child-free challenge our beliefs, so they're reviled.[272]

We also have a tendency to assume we know what's best for women. Those who stay childfree are told they're denying themselves the joys of motherhood. Without kids, we think women can never be truly happy.[273] One study looked at how we view women with and without children.[274] People thought "watching children grow up is life's greatest joy." They admitted it comes with responsibilities, but those are "labours of love." Women *want* to do these things for their families, we're told. On the other hand, the people in this study assumed women who stay childfree live lonely, meaningless lives. They thought these women must deeply regret their decision.

Not everyone thinks this way. Older people with less education are most likely to see child freedom as a bad thing.[275] These views are also more common in non-Western societies. But even in North America, older adults grew up with traditional beliefs about The Family. Today, they are parents or grandparents, and they badger their younger relatives, asking when they're going to have children of their own. Shock is common when their daughters say they want to stay childfree.

Often, these judgments are hurled at Millennials as a group. Older adults are often quick to tell Millennials to grow up. They criticize them for backpacking around Europe instead of getting a "real" job, marrying, and starting a family.[276] Millennials are seen as valuing an indulgent lifestyle—not the hard work and family values their parents want them to prioritize.[277]

These views are also stronger in some societies than others. In one study, Nigerians were asked what they thought of not having children.[278] In their culture, saying you don't want children is almost unheard of. Only monks and nuns willingly stay childfree. Many respondents talked about the risks of purposefully avoiding childbirth: namely, disgrace for themselves and their families. They said childfree women are seen as immoral, lazy, or even crazy. The majority didn't understand why anyone would choose not to have a family. As one woman put it: "there is no one on earth that does not want to have children."

Childfree women don't (always) feel lonely or full of regret. Many are happy to avoid the stress of trying to be a Good Mom.[279] They don't want to change their lifestyles or give up on their goals. Many say they value their freedom, independence, careers, and personal development. Motherhood, they believe, would interfere with all of these things.

What's more, some research shows that *mothers* are the unhappy ones. Having children can interfere with women's well-being.[280] To be Good Moms, they don't always have time to care for themselves. They're so focused on supporting their children, they struggle to meet their own needs. So, contrary to popular belief, motherhood doesn't guarantee happiness. Being a parent is only rewarding for people who find it rewarding.

With advances like the Pill, we like to think women are free to do as they please. But those who follow their own path come up against a great deal of judging. Women often stay childfree to hold on to their lives. That's why we call it "child freedom" instead of "childlessness": these women are making a positive decision to stay "free" from the responsibilities of parenthood. They don't see it as detracting from their quality of life.

That said, it takes a strong, confident woman to stand by this decision. These women know they'll be confronted harshly from all sides—likely, by their friends, family, and even their partners. That's enough to make many reconsider. In short, baby mania can convince even the least maternally inclined that they need children to be happy—or to save them from social ridicule.[281]

In fact, things might be getting a little worse, not better. Since 9/11, the Western world has felt vulnerable—not only to physical terrorist attacks, but to attacks on our culture as well.[282] Many feel as though their way of life and their beliefs are threatened. So they're throwing their support behind all things traditional. That includes beliefs in Good Moms, marriage, nuclear families, and so on.[283]

Nowhere is this clearer than in the U.S. There, a resurgence of traditional beliefs was reflected in the 2016 election of Donald Trump. For decades, the Western world was becoming more progressive: we were celebrating things like women in the workforce and gay marriage. But all the while, traditionalists have been mourning the loss of the beliefs they hold dear. This means two contrary things are going on. On the one hand, women are applauded for getting an education and growing their careers. But at the same time, they're also being shamed for being Bad Moms. By refusing to be stay at home moms, they're accused of doing themselves and their families an injustice.

For people who hold these traditional beliefs, women who regret having children are worst of all. These women are openly questioning the joys of motherhood. That means they could persuade other women not to have kids either. By shaming childfree women, traditionalists are trying to keep things the way they are. They're trying to hold on to the old-school beliefs they think are slipping through their fingers.

Infertility

Actively choosing to stay childfree is different than being unable to conceive. Women who *can't* have children are treated differently, and feel differently about their childlessness, than women who *choose* not to have children. Often, these women feel depressed and unfulfilled—the way we assume childfree women must feel.[284] Some of these feelings are caused by scrutiny and judgment from others. Not knowing about their infertility, many people assume these women are self-indulgent, crazy, or any of the other things childfree people are accused of being. Or they're told they should find a way around their "problem".[285] Fertility treatments are often seen as the "solution," even though they're expensive, invasive, and emotionally draining. But in our baby-obsessed society, people figure that anyone incapable of conceiving should do whatever it takes.

That says a lot about our views on fertility. If parenthood is normal, then infertility makes people abnormal. Some even see infertility as a disability: an impairment, or something "wrong."[286] Since we believe motherhood is the greatest thing a woman can achieve, those who can't conceive are seen as damaged.[287] After hearing these beliefs their entire lives, infertile women say they feel like they've "failed." They think their bodies have let them down, and feel incomplete. Without the family they planned for, these women feel desperate and isolated. They are *made* to feel that way by our beliefs, which make infertility out to be unwomanly and shameful.

Many infertile women are judged two times over. First, when they're in their prime childbearing years, they're asked why they don't have children yet. They are often criticized in the same way as willingly childfree women. Many only disclose their infertility to put a stop to these questions and unsolicited advice.[288] But then they're judged for their infertility. Whereas childfree women are often criticized loud and clear, infertile women are criticized much more subtly. Infertility is still taboo: women don't typically want to talk about it. When they do disclose it, many people feel uncomfortable—like they're prying into private matters. So, childfree women may have their choices and even their sanity openly questioned, but infertile women are more likely to be pitied. Those who *would* like to talk about their experiences often say they can't, thanks to this taboo.

Can Women Really Have It All?

One day, a staff member at a museum saw two unsupervised children making their way onto a ride. He announced over the PA system: "Where is the mother of these children?!"[289] At least two of our beliefs were voiced here. First, the ride attendant assumed the children's mother was taking them to the museum. (It could just as well have been their father.) Second, even if both parents were there, the attendant assumed the mother should be held accountable for leaving the kids unsupervised.

This shows the different responsibilities we believe men and women have. It also shows that people are willing to enforce those responsibilities. Throughout our lives, we watch men and women do different types of work.[290] We see moms feeding, clothing, changing, and chauffeuring their children around. In the meantime, dads clock long hours at the office, and maybe play with their children in the evening.[291] This arrangement is no longer a guarantee today, as more women work and more men help care for their kids. But it's still a familiar mold. Even if you didn't experience it yourself, you've seen this arrangement in movies and books, as I'll discuss in the next chapter. This traditional set up is so engrained in us, starting the moment we're born, it influences the ways women plan their lives.

As Sheryl Sandberg famously noted, these beliefs lead many women to self-sabotage their careers. Anticipating the demands of being a Good Mom, they turn down opportunities and scale back their responsibilities—even if they don't plan to have children for years.[292] On the other hand, men don't seem to think fatherhood will derail their careers. Unlike women, men ramp *up* their workload when they're planning to have kids. They seek promotions and raises so they can fill that breadwinning role we believe they should.

There's nothing wrong with scaling back at work to make time for family. Nor is there anything wrong with wanting a better-paying position to provide for that family. Problems arise when women and men feel pressured to make these popular choices.[293] For example, women shouldn't feel they must sacrifice their careers to become mothers.

Research shows that these beliefs affect the way we plan our future. Look at university students. One study found that students with higher career ambitions usually enjoyed successful, rewarding careers.[294] But, these high-achieving students typically said they wanted small families, or no children at all. On the other hand, many female students recognized they couldn't have it all. They said they'd like to get married and have kids, and maybe work part time on the side. These women also knew their choices would reinforce gender inequality. That is, they were aware their choices were traditional, and would keep alive the belief that women "should" stay at home with the children.

So, we can't blame parenthood itself for upholding the status quo. Rather, it's our beliefs about what it *means* to be a parent that make some women hold back at work. For the most part, these views are accurate: women dedicate more time to housework than men. And their responsibilities only increase after they have children.[295] Women are expected to care for their children and these efforts are rarely acknowledged. But men are praised for being involved in their children's lives at all. While women cook, clean, and chauffeur, men say they do the "optional" and fun activities, like helping with science projects or Boy Scouts.[296] And when they're out on family excursions together, women often take care of the practicalities—like booking tickets and packing snacks—while men get to play with their children and buy them presents.

In some families, women do get help. But that help often comes from other family members, like their own parents. Often, that means their husbands do even less of the work.[297] None of this is surprising: stay at home dads endure their fair share of stigma, told they're doing "women's work." Thus, many men shy away from the duties that would greatly help their wives, fearing they'll be made fun of.

Young women watch this happening all around them. They come to believe that motherhood consists of long days packing lunches, folding laundry, chauffeuring their children to soccer practice, and so on. Fifty years ago, this was "all" that people expected of women. It was still stressful, and there was still a learning curve when women had their first child. But for the most part, they weren't trying to juggle new motherhood with a career. Today, women are more likely than men to go to university (and more likely to get better grades). They are also dreaming of high status, high paying jobs. Yet, women are *also* expected to do all the motherly tasks women have always done.[298] Many young women know, before they've even made any WiSK decisions, that it will be too much to bear. In one study,[299] a 35-year-old woman named Ebony summarized: "Can you really be this established, awesome, tenured professor and be a wonderful parent and a loving and caring mate?"

Often, the answer is "no." Many women recognize their limits—physical, mental, and material—and must choose between a career and a family. It's bad enough that our beliefs keep women from fulfilling their dreams. But we're also setting the stage for the next generation.[300] If working women say they can't make room for a family, and mothers say they can't make room for a career, we're telling girls they *can't* have it all. They, too, will grow up to choose either a family *or* a career. They have few role models showing them how to do both.

The solution is more equally shared responsibilities at home. There's no reason for women to shoulder as much of the work as they do. Men are equally able to care for their children. Currently, we celebrate even the smallest contributions men make to childcare. But those contributions should be the rule, not the exception.[301] We need to change our expectations for fathers. Until we do, women's options in life will be limited.

The first step is recognizing the unequal responsibilities men and women have—and recognizing they are not compulsory. Men and women have filled different roles for centuries, but that's not a good reason to keep things the same. If you want a shot at having it all, you need to start today. Don't expect your partner to suddenly pitch in after your baby arrives and neither of you have slept in months. The responsibilities you have before kids predict the ones you'll have after kids. So, women who want to have children *and* a career should share responsibilities with their partners from the start—long before they start trying to conceive. That way, when the baby arrives, both partners will already be accustomed to sharing those responsibilities.

The Ticking Biological and Social Clocks

Geriatric pregnancy. Advanced maternal age. High-risk pregnancy.

This is how doctors describe pregnancy when you're over 35. True, it's harder for women to conceive as they age. And there are more risks for moms and fetuses alike. But these phrases highlight some of the negative views we have of older moms.

The growing number of women who are postponing childbearing are well aware. One study looked at women who had their first child at age 45.[302] These older mothers said others thought their experience was peculiar. One woman said she felt envious when she saw young couples with children. Another said she was embarrassed to be a first-time mother when her friends were becoming grandmothers.

These beliefs are part of the reason most women want to have children in their twenties or early thirties. Fifty-two percent of women say they want to have their first child when they're between 25 and 29.[303] Thirty-six percent want to wait until they're 30 to 34. As a woman in a different study put it: "it seems to have been so drilled into everyone's head that you know, without even thinking, you think 'oh I have to do it before 35'."[304]

In reality, both men and women have their first children when they're slightly older than they originally planned. Most Canadian women have their first child when they're between 30 and 34 years old.[305] But in the '70s and '80s, it was normal to have children in your early twenties. Today, 30 has become the new 20. That's how we know these beliefs are socially constructed, or collectively made up. People thought and behaved differently just a few decades ago. There's nothing "right" or necessary about having kids at a certain age. Most people just do what's expected of them.

Today, we expect women to have kids in a narrow window: not too old, but also not too young. Many bemoan their biological clocks, fearing their time for having children is running out.[306] But they also have "social clocks" to worry about. Certain social arrangements make it easier for some women to mother than others.[307] For example, single moms have it harder than mothers with partners in a lot of cases. One of the hardships single moms face is being judged by others. So, a single woman coming on forty may decide to have a baby by herself, to beat her biological clock. But that doesn't mean all her problems are solved. As a single, older mother, she'll probably face twice the stigma. People will question her decisions—"why would anyone *choose* single motherhood?"—and her parenting abilities—"she can't possibly be around enough to take good care of her child."

So, our biological clocks keep us from having kids when we're older, but our social ones keep us from having kids when we're young. Biologically, it would be best for women to have children in their twenties. But that's a terrible time, socially. Plenty of studies show women in their twenties feel that having a baby would derail their plans.[308] It would disrupt their education and career goals. Young women also worry they won't be able to financially support a child. And for the most part, we agree with them. Most people—young and old—believe women should be financially stable before starting a family.[309] In turn, as we know from earlier chapters, more women delay motherhood until their late twenties or early thirties.[310]

So, young women who say they are postponing childbearing do not face much stigma. It's "old" moms who get most of the heat. That means women only have a few years to have kids, if they want to avoid judgment.[311]

Final Thoughts

Sociologists study beliefs because we think they're functional. That is, beliefs are supposed to serve a purpose for us, as a society. For example, take the belief that people *should* become parents. We believe this because we need people to continue having children in order to survive as a species. If parenthood was shameful or embarrassing, far fewer women would be expecting.

Beliefs in Good Moms and Bad Moms are no different. We believe mothers should be selfless and love unconditionally because we want children to be safe and healthy. If we didn't have strong beliefs—and laws—about how children should be treated, abuse and neglect would be more widespread—or at least, more openly admitted. So, the popular beliefs we've discussed in this chapter can be useful. They can encourage people to start a scary new chapter of their lives: parenthood. They also help uphold high standards of childcare.

But some of these beliefs hurt more than they help. Most couples want and have children, so there's no need to shame those who don't. And women who try to be Good Moms can actually do damage to themselves and to their children. There's no such thing as a perfect pregnancy or a perfect parent. Women who feel pressured to be Good Moms end up burnt out and resentful of their children. And those children don't get the care they need from their exhausted mothers.

So, beliefs can be restrictive. They pressure people to conform, instead of letting them make their own decisions. Parenthood isn't some terrible thing that women need to be forced into; most look forward to it. More often, the beliefs we've discussed pressure women to take traditional paths through pregnancy, birth, and parenthood. They make it difficult for women to make different, less traditional choices—to stay childfree, for example. They also make women who aren't Good Moms feel ashamed and inadequate. In this sense, beliefs are the factor funnel itself. They shape all of our other considerations, swirling them around to produce our WiSK decisions. Without beliefs channeling our thoughts, people would be making much more diverse WiSK choices.

All of this is a little hypocritical, considering North Americans are proud of their "freedom." Here, women are supposed to be free to make their own decisions. Nothing good comes from shaming women who choose to stay childfree, or pitying women who can't have children. And, as we've said, burnout and inadequate child care are often the result when women try to be Good Moms.

Slowly but surely, women are starting to fight back. It's becoming clear that women cannot be the Good Moms our baby-maniacal society puts on a pedestal. More people are beginning to challenge the idea of a supermom. Whether it's a brave battle against PPD, an insistence on more equally shared childcare responsibilities, or the simple act of taking time for themselves, countless women are redefining what it means to be a Good Mom. In so doing, they're proving that popular beliefs don't define women or their worth. We have to support—not shame—women, so every individual can shape her own sense of self, whatever it may mean for her.

CHAPTER FIVE
Is Seeing Believing?
Parenthood in the Media

The last chapter showed people have a lot to say about pregnancy and parenthood. Beliefs shape the plans women make for their futures. But how are these beliefs spread? How do we learn them? And why do we (usually) feel pressured to conform to them? In this chapter, I look at one of the most powerful paths for spreading these beliefs: the media.

Representations of parenthood are everywhere. Gossip columnists are constantly on "bump patrol," speculating about which celebrities are expecting. Films and TV shows always have something to say about family; often, it's the plot's foundation. Books typically revolve around some sort of romance. Once you start thinking about it, the examples are endless. But we don't often think about it, because baby mania is commonplace. Dating, mating, and marriage are staples in every life course. So, they seep into all the media we consume, and we don't even realize it.

I talk about the media in two ways in this chapter. On one hand, the media *reflects* popular beliefs about parenthood. But on the other hand, it also *shapes* those views. The media is like a mirror: it reflects our society back to us. The people who create films, produce TV shows, write books, and write songs are influenced by the same beliefs as the rest of us. So, the media reflects the beliefs I discussed in the last chapter. But people also learn from the media. Depending on how they're depicted, we come to see certain behaviours as normal and others as strange after watching or reading about them. Most often, the media works in both of these ways at the same time. By reflecting beliefs that are already popular, the media keeps them alive.

However, this schema has two main problems. First, the number one goal of writers and producers is to attract the attention of viewers. That requires plotlines with shock value. No one wants to watch a movie that just shows a normal person going about her everyday business. Writers and producers know people want to see bizarre plots with lots of twists. *Jane the Virgin*, the parody telenovela I referenced earlier, is a good example. Jane, a 23-year-old Venezuelan-American virgin, gets pregnant when an alcoholic doctor accidentally artificially inseminates her with a sperm sample from her married boss, Rafael. Meanwhile, Rafael's former wife Petra splits her time sabotaging his business and trying to win Rafael back by inseminating herself with the rest of his sample. Oh, did I mention that Rafael's mother runs a drug ring? *Jane the Virgin* is obviously not a documentary-style depiction of everyday life. But, even this bizarre dramedy has important messages about parenthood, as we'll see below.

The second problem with this schema is that it's hard to know exactly how much the media influences the way we think or act. We absorb popular beliefs in a great many ways: from family, friends, and teachers, as well as media. So, there's no way to isolate the media as an independent variable. We can't prove that it—more than anything else—drives people to behave in certain ways—for example, to have children, or not have children, and so on.

That said, I do think the media plays a role in shaping our beliefs, no matter how small. According to data from 2013–14, Canadians age 18 to 34 watch an average of 20 hours of TV a week (Statistics Canada, 2015). In other words, young Canadians watch TV like it's their part-time job. Huge spans of our lifetimes are spent consuming media. These are the shows we binge watch with our friends, the movies we go out to see on dates, the magazines we read in the airport, and the novels we leaf through in bed each night. It would be silly to say they don't affect us at all. If they didn't engage us somehow—even if only as pure entertainment—we wouldn't spend most of our time watching and reading them. Everyone reacts to the media in one way or another: whether it's by agreeing with the beliefs depicted, striving to uphold them, questioning them, or rejecting them.

In sum, the media help shape our beliefs in many ways. But it would be impossible to analyze every piece of media that touches on parenthood. That would mean discussing just about all media content. Instead, my goal in this chapter is to look at just a handful of specific examples that construct motherhood, both positively and negatively, and in so doing, shape our beliefs. Once you start thinking about these implications, I'm willing to bet you can't stop.

Questions you'll get answers to:

▶ *How do these particular media pieces reflect popular beliefs about parenthood? How do they shape them?*

▶ *Judging from these media examples, what does a Good Mom look like? What about a Bad Mom? How do these beliefs impact women's WiSK decisions? How do they play into feelings of shame, fear, and guilt?*

▶ *How have some media challenged those stereotypes? Where do we see the media applauding moms who don't conform to tradition?*

▶ *How might some media make moms feel about themselves? How might they influence women who are thinking about becoming moms?*

▶ *How have these media examples challenged myths about abortion?*

▶ *Why don't we see many permanently infertile women in the media?*

Celebrity Super Moms: Setting Impossibly High Standards

Make-up free Reese Witherspoon picks up youngest son Tennessee from his karate lesson in Brentwood. This October 2017 *Daily Mail* article praises the actor for "attending to her motherly duties." It goes on: "When she's not on set, she is taking care of her beautiful three children." Paparazzi photos show Witherspoon—wearing heels and a top from her own couture line—escorting her uniform-clad five-year-old home from karate.

Super soccer mom! Denise Richards displays her impressive pitching skills as she fields an errant ball during daughter Lola's game. Even while carrying a blanket and cooler of post-practice snacks, Richards looks like a Barbie in yoga pants: "Denise Richards proved ever the supportive and doting mom as she took daughter Lola to soccer practice on Thursday in Beverly Hills."

Five celebrity parents who get their own groceries. "With her re-usable shopping bags in tow, Jessica Alba is often seen getting groceries with her daughters, Honor, 4, and Haven, 1, at Whole Foods in Los Angeles."

These are all boringly normal chores every parent does. Yet, when celebrities do them, they're headline-worthy. These are the people we build up in our minds to be larger than life: with their perfect hair/teeth/legs/husbands/houses/children, we imagine celebrities living glamorous, lavish lives. Because we idolize celebrities like this, it seems strange to see them doing the same things "normal" moms do. They must be constantly preoccupied, we think to ourselves, with whatever it is celebrities do: rehearsing, filming, recording, signing contracts, walking the red carpet, getting glammed up to walk that red carpet, and being annoyed by paparazzi in their faces every time they set foot outside. But then we see photographic proof that they *also* make time to chat with the other soccer moms. What's more, they never forget to bring reusable bags to pack their organic veggies in. They're always on time to pick up their children from karate lessons—while modelling the latest top from their own couture line. It seems these celebrity Super Moms have figured out how to Have It All.

If these famous women can balance motherhood with the highest-profile careers imaginable, there's no excuse for the rest of us.[312] If Denise Richards can find the time to watch her daughter's soccer game—looking like a perfectly toned yet effortlessly casual Barbie, no less—then why can't you? What's your excuse for feeding your children pizza for the second night in a row when Jessica Alba can keep two children in check while perusing pesticide-free produce?

The reality is that these women have infinitely more resources than working-class and even middle-class moms. Maybe Richards' nanny prepped and packed that cooler full of snacks for her. And maybe Alba's driver is chauffeuring them to and from the grocery store. Sometimes, cleverly cropped photos make women look like Super Moms by keeping their nannies and childcare workers just outside of the frame.[313]

Sure, celebrities are people too. Hurray for those of them who cheer their children on from the soccer field sidelines, and bring them along to do the grocery shopping. Witherspoon, Richards, and Alba look like great moms, and they deserve to be portrayed as such in the media. Problems only arise when the rest of us take them as a standard of comparison: when we start thinking, *if they can do it, I should be able to too.*

These comparisons are dangerous because they're unattainable. Though *People* magazine says celebrities are just like us, the truth is, they're not. At least, not when it comes to parenting. Being a parent is draining in every sense of the word: it drains your money, time, and energy. With bottomless wallets, celebrities can pay to make parenthood work for them. They can afford live-in nannies, housekeepers, private tutors, chauffeurs, and more. For the remaining 99 percent of us, these luxurious helpers are out of reach. Yet, despite their different resources, these unfathomably wealthy women are depicted as a standard for how comparatively poor women are supposed to mother.[314]

Inevitably, regular moms fail to live up to these impossibly high standards. Seeing glamorous celebrities effortlessly juggle the exact same tasks only makes them feel worse. A second night of pizza for dinner becomes all the more guilt-inducing when you see Alba making time for her Whole Foods run. And when the babysitter picks your kid up from ballet because you're working late, it doesn't feel great to see Witherspoon "attending to her motherly duties" in heels and frills.

This self-shaming can start before a child is even born. Gossip rags were practically invented for photo galleries of celebrities' pre- and post-baby bodies: "After giving birth to Prince George in July 2013, [Kate] Middleton looked enviably thin right away, and a source told *Us* she had 'hardly done anything to lose the weight.' 'Kate's still breastfeeding and the small weight she gained while pregnant has just melted off,' the insider said. 'She's not dieting'".[315] Another article titled "Fit Moms We Love" applauds Halle Berry: "This 44-year-old mom uses kickboxing, intervals and a healthy diet to stay so trim and toned. Talk about a healthy example for her family!"[316]

The endless photos, weight loss "secrets," workout challenges, and words of wisdom from celebrities who instantly lose their baby weight put the spotlight on new moms' bodies.[317] Women like Berry who shed the pounds are glorified as great role models for their children. Meanwhile, we're supposed to envy Middleton, who barely gained weight while pregnant and didn't have to put in any effort to get rid of it post-baby. Just like pizza-reliant mom feels guilty seeing Alba in Whole Foods, so too do moms who hold on to their mummy tummy after giving birth—that is, every single mother, ever. Without a personal trainer pushing them through tough workouts and a private chef whipping up nutritious low-calorie meals, most moms take about a year to get back to their pre-pregnancy weight, if they ever do. Applauding celebrities for losing huge amounts of weight mere weeks after giving birth just makes regular moms feel bad about themselves. *If they can do it, I should be able to too*, we think.

On the flip side, there are also those celebrities the media loves to hate. The media shame those who hold on to their baby weight for a few months, for example: not only are they made fun of for being fat, but they're also made out to be Bad Moms.[318] If they can't keep their own bodies under control, how are they supposed to care for their newborn?

For many moms, these expectations are impossibly high. It's hard enough to adjust after giving birth, especially if you're a first-time mom. Now, besides all the criteria for good mothering I outlined in the last chapter—unconditional love, self-sacrificing devotion—you also have to be a size two within a few months of giving birth.[319] We've taken the idea of a Supermom to a whole new level. It's no wonder that so many women, questioning if they can really Have It All, are delaying parenthood for longer and longer.

The Terrifying Bad Mom: Horror Film Tropes

The multi-billion-dollar horror film industry was built on freaking people out. Scary movies are meant to tap into our deepest, darkest fears. For Bad Moms to feature so prominently in these films says a lot about what we, as a society, are most afraid of.

Consider just two of these films: Lynne Ramsay's *We Need to Talk about Kevin* (2011) and Jennifer Kent's *The Babadook* (2014). Both do what horror movies are supposed to: they make viewers scared and uncomfortable. This they do by focusing attention on Bad Moms who shatter our idealized notions of parenthood. Viewers find themselves vilifying these Bad Moms: women who resent—even hate—their own children. You aren't just scared of these moms for the sake of their kids; you're scared that you too could become a monster if you ever became a parent.

In *We Need to Talk about Kevin*, protagonist Eva tries to rebuild her life after a terrible tragedy. Her son, Kevin, has perpetrated a school shooting, and murdered her husband and daughter. The film shows present-day Eva living in isolation, working an unfulfilling job, and occasionally visiting Kevin in prison. But in flashbacks to the past, we see Eva's memories of Kevin's childhood. From the moment he was born, Kevin's relationship with Eva has been strained. He cries only with her, never with his father; he refuses to play games; and he destroys everything she loves. Every memory Eva has of Kevin makes her feel he was always purposely defying her.

The Babadook follows Amelia's struggle to raise her son Samuel. Amelia's husband died in a car crash while racing Amelia to the hospital to give birth. So, Amelia associates Samuel with her husband's death. Amelia and Samuel are tormented throughout the film by the Babadook: a materialization of her depression. It begins by making her exhausted, so she struggles to meet her son's demands. But Amelia is eventually consumed by the Babadook, and she unleashes her untapped resentment towards her son. While Amelia blames Samuel for her sleepless nights, pain, and isolation, Samuel tries to both fight and protect his mother. The film ends with Amelia finally locking the Babadook in the basement. She can never be free from the trauma that will haunt her for the rest of her life, but she has promised to keep it from hindering her relationship with Samuel.

Eva and Amelia become villains in these stories because they aren't Good Moms. They don't put their child's needs above their own; they don't love unconditionally; they don't accept their child's failings; and they certainly don't stay calm and patient.[320] In one of Eva's flashbacks, Kevin purposefully soils himself and tries to force Eva to clean him. She accidentally breaks his arm in response. In another scene, she snaps when Kevin glares at her in silence instead of passing her a ball: "Mommy was happy before little Kevin came along, did you know that? Now Mommy wakes up every morning and wishes she was in France!" Eva is far from a calm, composed Good Mom.

Few people could keep it together while trying to deal with a child as difficult as Kevin. Yet many viewers still think Eva is evil. Some even blame her for Kevin's horrific crimes. In the comments section of the film's trailer on YouTube, one viewer wrote: "What we really need to pay attention [to] is not the fact that Kevin is a creepy psychopath, but what makes Kevin such a monster. It's his MOTHER."[321] Another comment reads: "I actually thought she was a terrible mother, it's like she never wanted him even as a baby. She didn't hold him properly or show any love to him whatsoever. I think she has psychopathic tendencies, she's so cold and hard. He's like her and it seems like everything he does is to emotionally destroy her, it all seems to be targeted at her. He is a psychopath but I think she contributed to it a great deal."[322]

So, Bad Moms like Eva are to blame for their children's terrifying actions. We see this reflected in the film itself: Eva is routinely attacked by people who attribute her son's murders to her bad mothering. Her home gets drenched in red paint, someone breaks her eggs in the grocery store, and she even gets slapped. Eva's neighbours hold her responsible for the shooting and don't think she deserves happiness, or even peace. But Eva also holds *herself* responsible. She never stands up for herself, and even says she knows she's going straight to hell. In sum, Eva is the ultimate villain, and it's because she's a Bad Mom.

Amelia is vilified for the same reasons. Once the Babadook takes over, Amelia doesn't have a shred of patience left. She starts mocking Samuel and cuts the phone line so he can't call anyone for help. In the film's most off-putting scene, she belittles him for wetting himself and says: "You don't know how many times I wished it was you and not him that died."

What's terrifying about *The Babadook* is its depiction of maternal apathy and even spite.[323] Amelia horrifies us because she doesn't have any maternal instincts. Good Moms are nurturing, tender, and compassionate—and Amelia is none of these things. Even before she's possessed by the evil Babadook, Amelia doesn't express love or affection for her son. She doesn't want to be a mom. So it's not the cartoonish monster that makes *The Babadook* a horror film; it's the "unnatural" Bad Mom who doesn't love her own kid.

Eva and Amelia are also terrifying in another sense. They frighten the many women who fear they too will live through these nightmares. Eva and Amelia bring to life the many worries women have about their own mothering abilities. And they challenge the fantasy that motherhood is pure, easy bliss.

We know from the previous chapter that plenty of women have concerns about becoming moms. They worry that, to be a Good Mom, they'll have to give up some of their own hopes and dreams. And then these women see Eva: the only scene in the entire film where she seems happy is when she's in Spain, working as a travel writer—before she's pregnant. Her heart breaks when she has to move from New York City into the suburbs, where her husband insists that Kevin can have a better childhood. Kevin then proceeds to ruin everything Eva loves, including her special room in their new house, which he destroys with a paint gun. And once her son—whom she's changed so much for—commits mass murder, everyone thinks *she* should suffer for the rest of her life. So, *We Need to Talk about Kevin* turns women's nightmares of self-sacrifice into realities.

Similarly, *The Babadook* shows how some women lose

themselves entirely when they become moms. Most women who are seriously considering having children expect sleepless months, constant demands for attention, and even some frustration and disappointment. But watching Amelia struggle makes you wonder if those challenges are worth it. Amelia's constantly exhausted and consumed by mothering. Hesitant future moms aren't reassured that they have what it takes to raise a child.

Finally, both films shatter the comforting idea that mothering is instinctive: something that comes naturally to all women.[324] Instead, *We Need to Talk about Kevin* and *The Babadook* show that motherhood can be lonely and depressing. Watching these films, we realize that a mother's love isn't guaranteed: it's something that mothers can give or withdraw, or may never materialize.[325] That realization taps into our deepest fears. What if you have a baby and don't love it? What if, like Eva, giving birth is miserable, instead of joyful and fulfilling? What if all the sleepless nights and temper tantrums *aren't* worth it in the end? What if motherhood isn't blissful—what if it makes you sick with depression and worse off than you were before? Eva and Amelia are (fictional) living proof of the terrifying possibility that children can be born to Bad Moms—and that you yourself could become one of them.

Fictional Fears Brought to Life

Some true crime TV shows, documentaries, and podcasts make these horror-film-induced fears feel very real. One popular sub-genre shocks and horrifies viewers by showing children suffering in part because they have Bad Parents. In this section, I look at just two of the hundreds of pieces of media that can make the thought of becoming a parent absolutely terrifying: documentaries focusing on pedophilia.

First, *Leaving Neverland* (2019) was one of the most-watched documentaries on HBO. In it, two men now in their thirties allege that celebrity Michael Jackson sexually abused them when they were children. Their mothers Joy and Stephanie feature just as prominently in the documentary, recalling how Jackson befriended them decades ago, and how they were manipulated into making such poor parenting decisions. The men themselves have received mixed reactions, with many offering support and sympathy, and others accusing them of lying to win Jackson's wealth in court. But the majority agree that, if the allegations are true, it's the victims' mothers we should be blaming. In 2013, when Wade Robson filed a lawsuit against Jackson, a TMZ staffer said: "He should sue his mom for letting him go sleep with Michael Jackson when he was 7 years old."[326] When allegations from others surfaced years earlier, one columnist wrote that parents who brought their children to the star's Neverland Ranch "should be investigated and possibly prosecuted themselves".[327]

Joy and Stephanie are right up there with Eva and Amelia, vilified as the ultimate Bad Moms. The difference is, it's possible these horrors happened in real life. And that means they could happen to you, too. So, Eva and Amelia tap into one kind of fear: the horror that you might not love your own kid. But Joy and Stephanie tap into yet another kind: what if your child suffers immeasurably, and you are partly to blame?

Second, Netflix documentary *Abducted in Plain Sight* makes a similar point. Immediately infatuated with 12-year-old Jan Broberg, 40-year-old Robert Berchtold spends years befriending her parents, Mary Ann and Bob, so he can spend time with her. He didn't just make sure they trusted him around their kids; he tricked them *both* into developing sexual relationships with him. So when Berchtold took Jan "horseback riding" and never brought her home, her parents didn't contact the FBI for days—and even then, they remained convinced that this man they both cared for would never hurt her. It took years and Jan's second abduction by Berchtold before the truth finally came out: he had drugged, molested, and raped her an estimated 200 times.

The documentary has been met with sheer disbelief. Mary Ann and Bob have (arguably) come under even more fire than Joy and Stephanie. And though all four of these parents try to explain the web of manipulation, deceit, and even blackmail that led to their poor decisions, not one makes excuses for what happened. The Brobergs say they were so honest about their humiliating experiences because they don't want other families to suffer like they did. What's terrifying, then, is that there's a need for this sort of cautionary tale in the first place. The true crime genre shows potential parents some of the most disturbing fates their future children could suffer. These documentaries point to just one kind of horrifying danger that could wrack their families with guilt and shame for the rest of their lives. The other factors we've discussed throughout this book—from financial instability, to unfulfilled career goals, to less-than-ideal living arrangements—are scary enough for people who aren't sure if they want to become parents. Media that get us thinking about all the other potential threats make that future plain terrifying.

Watching Mothers Mother

The opening scene of *Knocked Up* shows just how different Alison and Ben's lives are, before they have a child. Ben fills his days with pot, roller coasters, and porn. Alison, on the other hand, is up at the crack of dawn, getting ready for another day at the job she loves, and dropping her nieces off at school. The implication is clear: women are naturally responsible caregivers, destined to be Good Moms. Men, by contrast, need some prodding. So when Alison finds herself pregnant with Ben's baby after a one-night stand, we never think Ben will become a single dad. If the pair can't make parenthood work together, we automatically assume Alison will go it alone. After all, she's the only viable parent material.

Films like *Knocked Up* make us laugh because they poke fun at our beliefs. It's fun to watch Seth Rogan mess everything up, and see how much it annoys uptight Katherine Heigl. Though good natured, these kinds of characters reinforce some stereotypes. They paint women as the rule-enforcing killjoys who will become helicopter moms. Meanwhile, men are shown as the fun-loving goofballs their children want to play with. The characters are only funny because we know exactly the types of people they're making fun of.

In reality though, parents come in all different shapes and sizes. And some media do a great job of showing just how diverse parents are. Take *Jane the Virgin* as an example. Despite its bizarre plot, many characters on this show are mothers, and no two are exactly alike.

First, we have the deeply religious grandmother, Alba, and her sexually adventurous daughter, Xiomara. These two characters represent age-old archetypes of motherhood: the Virgin Madonna and the Whore. Psychoanalyst Sigmund Freud is often credited with inventing this idea. He said some of his male patients thought of women like this: they were either saintly, chaste Madonnas, or debased whores. These men loved their wives, who they saw as Madonnas; but they weren't sexually attracted to them because they respected them too much. Instead, they lusted after women they saw as whores: promiscuous women they thought were obsessed with sex.

Freud called this the Madonna/Whore dichotomy. By "dichotomy," he meant our inability to reconcile the two. Women are put in one of these boxes, categorized as an untouched Girl Next Door, *or* a sex-crazed prostitute. There's no middle ground.

Alba and Xiomara are good examples of this Madonna/Whore dichotomy. With her stuffy clothing, ever-present rosary, and lectures about the sanctity of marriage, Alba is a model Madonna. Xiomara's character contrasts sharply: she's a seductress who isn't afraid to show off her curves. They share their different outlooks on sex in the very first scene of *Jane the Virgin*. Ten-year-old Jane stands in her bedroom with a white flower in her hand. Alba tells her, "Look at the flower in your hand, Jane. Notice how perfect it is. How pure. Now *mija*, crumple it up." Xiomara interrupts from where she's sitting on Jane's bed, wearing a denim jumpsuit that shows a lot of leg and a lot of cleavage: "Really, mom?" she whines. "Shh!" chides Alba. "But this is so lame!" Xiomara scowls, painting her nails.

Jane sides with her grandmother. She gets boxed into the Virgin category when she shows her fascination with Alba's exercise, telling her mom to be quiet and crumpling the flower in her palm. "Now try to make it look new again," Alba instructs Jane (as Xiomara rolls her eyes, remembering when she did the same experiment when she was Jane's age). "I can't," says Jane, and Alba sternly replies: "That's right. You can never go back. And that's what happens when you lose your VIRGINITY." (Cue more eye-rolling from Xiomara.)

So, in scene one of episode one, Alba and Xiomara are cast as the Madonna and the Whore of *Jane the Virgin*. Plenty of media—especially older films—have been criticized for boxing female characters into these categories. *Jane the Virgin* stands out because it questions this dichotomy and gives us alternatives. Take Petra: Jane's frenemy, and Rafael's first wife. Petra's certainly sexy; the narrator introduces her as a "man-eater" after we watch her trying to help her husband "relax." But as the show progresses, we start to see Petra's soft side: she becomes a single mom of twins, struggles with post-partum depression, and learns how to make motherhood work for her. All the while, she's clawing her way up the corporate ladder and struggling to shake her troubled past.

There's also Jane. No one fits the Madonna archetype better than a pregnant virgin. Yet Jane's desire for not one but two men shows us that even the most innocent, naïve-looking women have sex drives too. Like Petra, Jane refuses to let motherhood steamroll her career. She overcomes countless obstacles to writing her novel and even pursues grad school, all with her baby boy Mateo in tow.

So, *Jane the Virgin* does play into the Madonna/Whore dichotomy, like so many shows before it. But it also depicts female characters who don't fit these stereotypes. As Jane and Petra show, there's more to mothers than their chastity or promiscuity. Mothers can also have jobs, relationships, goals, work ethics, and lives. In sum, the show validates many different kinds of mothers, each with their own values, challenges, and parenting strategies. What it does not do is preach an ideal of what a mother "should" be.

Better still, *Jane the Virgin* shows men doing "women's work." It also makes the case that non-nuclear families can function just fine. When Jane first realizes she's pregnant, she considers giving the baby to Rafael and Petra. She assumes the baby would have two loving parents who fit the traditional family mould. But when Jane learns Rafael and Petra are thinking about getting a divorce, she questions keeping her baby altogether. Alba's religiosity has rubbed off on her, and Jane thinks only happily married couples should have children. The show traces Jane's journey from this common, conservative belief, to her eventual realization that a baby doesn't need a traditional nuclear family to be happy and healthy. When Mateo is born, he splits his time between Rafael, Jane, Michael, Xiomara, Alba, and Jane's dad, Rogelio. Everyone pitches in, making for one big support system that raises Mateo collectively. Seeing this unorthodox arrangement on TV makes it seem more normal.

We see the same mix of picture-perfect and more realistic depictions of motherhood on social media. On the one hand, you have hundreds of Instagram accounts that make babies look like glam accessories, toted around by beautifully made-up mothers who are forever on vacation or lounging in their living rooms that look like they're straight out of magazines. Amanda Stanton from ABC's *The Bachelor* is just one example. Her profile features photos almost exclusively of herself looking like a supermodel, with perfectly tousled hair and elaborate outfits, alongside her two girls who are almost always playing with toys or wearing clothes that Amanda's been paid to promote to her followers. Her fellow *Bachelor* contestants Carly Waddell and Evan Bass also make new parenthood look easy and use their social media accounts to model the latest baby accessories. Just like the anxiety-inducing tabloids I talked about earlier, these social profiles can make average moms wonder why they're having such a hard time keeping up. *If Amanda and Carly can always put on make-up and do their hair, I should be able to too.*

But on the other hand, there's also a groundswell of women pushing back against the idea that mothers have to make it seem like they always have their lives perfectly together. Many "mommy bloggers" make it their mission to be real and relatable. For example, Jennifer van Huss, the mom behind blog "1 Heart, 1 Family," explains: "I am by no means the perfect mother, but I feel through my mistakes, hurdles and occasional triumphs, other moms will learn that they are not alone!" Another Canadian mom named Lisa Thornbury shares what it's like to raise a daughter with a disability on her blog "Forever in Mom Genes." She realizes that, though her experiences may be different from other mothers', they're equally worth photographing and writing about. And "The Rebel Mama" bloggers Aleks and Nikita say they want to help more people see "that there is more than one formula for a healthy family dynamic *and more than one kind of woman who can be a good mom.*"

So, while social media can shame women for "failing" to live up to Good Mom expectations, it can also help them feel like they aren't alone in the daily struggles of parenting. Some accounts may help people thinking about starting a family realize that, as tough as it can be, motherhood is also often rewarding.

Can Good Moms Have Careers?

Grey's Anatomy is another TV show that challenges convention. Most of the leading characters are Ivy League-educated female surgeons who work 80-hour weeks and put their careers first. Work/life balance is always being commented on.

Plenty of scenes show husbands pressuring their wives to work less and mother more. Fan-favourite Miranda Bailey's marriage eventually fell apart because her husband, Tucker, couldn't handle her long shifts at the hospital. Time and again, he questioned whether Miranda was even "interested in being part of this family." Tucker's constant criticism eventually makes even strong-willed Miranda internalize some beliefs about Good Moms. In one episode, Miranda blames herself when her son has an accident while she is at work. She thinks it's her fault because a Good Mom would be there to protect her child.

That even Miranda can be made to feel guilty shows just how strong our belief in the Good Mom is. But, rather than showing Miranda trying to uphold this image, *Grey's Anatomy* encourages us to empathize with her. We know and love Miranda for being an amazing life-saving surgeon, and the glue that holds the rest of the cast together. We *want* her to prioritize her career, and we know she can keep saving lives while also being a great mom.

In this sense, *Grey's Anatomy's* greatest strength is also one of its weaknesses. Miranda is the epitome of a woman who Has It All. At the peak of her career, she remarries, gets promoted to Chief of Surgery, and even manages the drama of shared custody. Her character reassures women that they can succeed in prestigious jobs while still being happily married Good Moms. It's an empowering message that's inspired many. At the same time, though, Miranda might set the bar unreasonably high. Like celebrity Super Moms—who lose their baby weight in weeks, always shop organic, and pick their children up from karate wearing heels—Miranda is exceptional. Juggling so many demanding roles isn't realistic for most people.

So, while *Grey's Anatomy* applauds successful working moms, some women would be unhappy and unhealthy if they tried to be like Miranda. Feelings of guilt or self-doubt might seep in as yet another piece of media making women think, *If she can do it, I should be able to too.*

Meredith Grey, *Grey's Anatomy's* leading lady, may ease some of these fears. She dreads turning into her own mother: a brilliant surgeon but neglectful mom. Meredith's husband, Derek Sheppard, occasionally makes off-hand remarks that feed her insecurities. For example, in the seventh season, when Meredith frets over all the "mom" chores she doesn't know how to do, like making lunches and Halloween costumes, Derek replies: "Good moms make Halloween costumes."

Comments like that go to show how arbitrarily we define Good Moms. Whether you hand-sew your daughter's princess costume or pick one up at the dollar store has little impact on the fun she has trick-or-treating. Think about just how many moms *don't* make their children Halloween costumes. Each of these women falls outside of Derek's definition of a Good Mom. When you think about all of these off-hand remarks, made in all different types of media, they start to add up. And when women don't live up to the high standards set by these fictional characters, they come to feel they've failed their children.

Grey's Anatomy paints sympathetic portraits of women who battle these insecurities. It shows how much a seemingly innocent comment can hurt—especially for women who are already anxious about mothering. And, when characters like Meredith eventually overcome their fears and become Good Moms in their own way, the show provides hope for women who are questioning if they have what it takes.

Saying "No" to the Motherhood Mandate

In yet another one of the moving monologues that made *Grey's Anatomy* famous, Arizona Robbins lets her girlfriend, Callie Torres, have it: "I'm not broken. I'm not some psycho trauma. My lack of interest in having a child is not some pathology that you can pat yourself on the back for having diagnosed. I like my life. I like it the way it is" (*Grey's Anatomy*, Season 6, Episode 20).

Callie desperately wants to have a baby, and can't understand why Arizona—a paediatric surgeon who spends her days caring for children who adore her—wouldn't want a child of her own. Her mindset is a popular one. As I discussed in the last chapter, many see having children as an inevitable step in the life course. So, Callie assumes something about motherhood is scaring Arizona—that there's something "wrong" with her that they can identify and fix. When Callie learns that Arizona's brother died when they were young, she celebrates having discovered her trigger. Arizona must be scared that, just like her own parents, she too would risk losing her child. After all, she takes care of desperately ill children, and watches many of them die. When Callie "diagnoses" Arizona with this fear, Arizona launches into her tirade.

Yet again, *Grey's Anatomy* shows how the people we love— even progressive, open-minded people—can reinforce traditional beliefs. Even Callie, who fights back against stigmatization on the show, is here guilty of assuming that all women want children, no matter how fiercely they deny it. This assumption is known as the "motherhood mandate": the expectation that every woman will eventually become a mother.[328] But when Arizona comes out on top with her strong, confident monologue, she's showing women who don't want to have children—at all, ever—that their choice is valid too. There's nothing "wrong" with them, no problem that needs to be "diagnosed" or past trauma that needs to be "fixed." Rather, both Callie *and* Arizona's outlooks are valid. Some women will be excited to be moms and others will live happy, fulfilled lives without children.

Another couple on the show, Christina Yang and Owen Hunt, also have opposing beliefs. Like Callie, Owen thinks parenthood is an inevitable step in the life course. He accuses his wife of being childish when she insists she doesn't want children, and never will. "The idea that your career is the only thing that will ever matter ... is, frankly, a young person's notion," he tells her. "You're gonna change your mind in three years or five and then it's gonna be too late and you're gonna regret it," he goes on.[329]

Both Callie and Owen are deeply hurt that their partner is denying them their dream of becoming parents. The problem is that neither Callie nor Owen realizes that they are hurting their partners in exactly the same way by expecting them to "come around."[330] They think their vision of the future is the only desirable one: that they alone are the normal people who deserve empathy, while their partners are disturbed victims or immature Millennials.

Grey's Anatomy suggests people like Arizona and Christina deserve to be heard too. That's why there's so much dialogue insisting "it's alright to never want children."[331] The show points out that people who want children are assumed to have valid reasons, but those who don't are always being asked to justify their choice, or cautioned that they'll regret it. Instead of shaming these women, *Grey's Anatomy* makes us see their side of things.

No Regrets: Challenging Abortion Myths

Like all good primetime shows, *Grey's Anatomy* keeps pumping Christina and Owen's marriage full of drama. In season 7, when they find out Christina's pregnant, she doesn't budge: "I don't want one. I don't hate children, I respect children; I think they should have parents who *want* them...." Owen insists: "*I* want them ... I could take a [paternity] leave ... It doesn't have to be your problem, it'll be my problem. You wouldn't even—" "What, *notice?*" Christina cuts him off. "I'm not a monster. If I have a baby I'll love it." "That's a problem we can work with," Owen laughingly replies.

Their argument highlights the ways people—including and sometimes especially the ones we love most—can belittle the choice to stay childfree. Owen laughs at this choice and reduces it to a scheduling issue. All the while, he can't see that some of his own suggestions are ridiculous. Insisting Christina's life wouldn't change at all if they were to have the baby just goes to show how little Owen knows about parenthood.

Meredith, Christina's best friend, tells him as much. She warns him: "the guilt of resenting her own kid will eat her alive." Meredith's monologue refutes some of the pro-life beliefs I discussed earlier. Namely, it's often said that most women regret having abortions. But Meredith points out that following through on an unwanted pregnancy can also cause huge regret and emotional pain, both for the mother and the child. She tells Owen that forcing Christina to go through with this "will almost kill her … [and] it will almost kill your kid."[332] Ultimately, Owen realizes he needs to support Christina's decision to have an abortion. Though he looks heartbroken and disappointed, he holds Christina's hand as the procedure begins.

Grey's Anatomy also makes a point of highlighting the secrecy and shame that often surround abortion. Owen and Christina's relationship gradually disintegrates in the aftermath. They refuse to speak about the procedure, referring to the abortion as "it." This is not to say that abortions ruin marriages. Rather, it shows that the *stigma* surrounding abortion—and the stigma around the choice to stay childfree—persists. Maybe, if they had felt comfortable talking openly about their choices and actions, Owen and Christina would still be together.

Fast forward four years to 2015. Olivia Pope, leading lady of hit show *Scandal*, gets about one minute of airtime devoted to her abortion.[333] We don't even know she's pregnant until we see her enter a doctor's office, don a gown and cap, and stretch out on an operating table for a minimally invasive procedure. Olivia's abortion certainly doesn't steal the show; it's a subplot, at best. And when it's over, she just moves on with her life.

Much like Christina, Olivia challenges the idea that getting an abortion is always a painful, life-altering decision. We don't see either of them tearfully weighing their options, or having tormented discussions with their partners, trying to figure out what to do. True, Christina argues relentlessly with Owen, but only because she is so sure of her choice. And Olivia doesn't even tell her partner about the abortion. We certainly never see them regret their choice or wonder, "what if?"

Abortion scenes like Christina's and Olivia's are rare in mainstream media. Networks don't want to risk offending viewers and send their ratings plummeting by depicting something taboo. So, it was no surprise when Shonda Rhymes, creator of both *Grey's Anatomy* and *Scandal*, said her network "freaked out a bit" when she pitched Christina's abortion storyline. Because there was no real precedent, ABC pressured Rhymes to change Christina's story. And long-time fans will remember that, in the first season, instead of having an abortion, an unexpectedly pregnant Christina conveniently miscarries.[334] It took seven years before Rhymes was finally given the go-ahead to show Christina and Owen holding hands during the procedure in season 8.

But she didn't have an easy time getting Olivia's abortion on air either. This time, it was 2015, and ABC once again told Rhymes they wanted to cut the scene.[335] Rhymes and some of the cast made a fuss, insisting they would splash the cut all over the news—so it went ahead.

Of course, airing a few abortion scenes doesn't mean the procedure is widely accepted all of a sudden. Maybe Christina and Olivia's scenes changed the minds of a few pro-lifers. More likely, it caused the same backlash and outrage I discussed in an earlier chapter. That's why we're even talking about their abortions in this book at all: these were controversial decisions for a mainstream network. That many people found the scenes unacceptable shows just how far we still have to go. Think about it: millions of viewers watch TV shows like *Game of Thrones*, where pornographic sex scenes are commonplace, or *The Walking Dead*, where more skulls are crushed than words are spoken. Yet a minute-long scene showing a woman in stir-rups is considered newsworthy and scandalous.

Nevertheless, by putting abortion in the spotlight, shows like *Grey's Anatomy* and *Scandal* have taken an important step. They show smart, successful, well-liked women gaining sympathy and approval for what some might call taboo decisions. These depictions comfort the many women who make similar decisions, but are told those decisions are bad or strange. Seeing these stories on TV normalizes them in reality. So, while we may have a long way to go, it's only by openly talking about abortion that we'll be able to make it an acceptable choice.

Jane the Virgin does a good job of maintaining that open-mindedness. It shows that *everyone* has something to say when it comes to a woman's right to choose. When she discovers she's pregnant, Jane is bombarded with conflicting advice. Her mother makes it clear that she would support Jane's choice to abort, because she doesn't think Jane should throw away her education and career. Jane's Catholic grandmother unsurprisingly encourages her to keep the baby. Jane's fiancé Michael, though mostly supportive, puts a little pressure on her to abort; he's not excited about starting their life together raising another man's child. Finally, Rafael and Petra desperately want Jane to continue the pregnancy; she conceived using (what they initially thought was) Rafael's last sperm sample.

We know Jane ultimately decides to keep the baby—and she makes that decision independently and self-assuredly. But the sheer number of conflicting opinions that are thrown at her show people aren't afraid to make a woman's pregnancy their business. No one knows that better than the real women who choose to have abortions—and publicly share the experience. From books like *Shout Your Abortion*—which compiles essays, photos, and creative projects that have helped women talk about their decisions on their own terms—to popular publications like *The Huffington Post* that devote entire sections to opinion pieces on abortion, the media landscape is flooded with content that helps shape our beliefs on the pro-choice versus pro-life debate.

Ghosts of Primetime: Indefinitely Infertile Women

When Meredith Grey finally decides she's ready to get pregnant, she can't. She suffers a miscarriage, then struggles to conceive again. Ultimately, she turns to fertility clinics and drugs in the hopes that they will soothe her supposedly "hostile uterus."

Just as it challenged abortion myths, *Grey's Anatomy* does a great job of busting some infertility myths too. Meredith hilariously frets that she can't conceive for a number of reasons—from her college-era tequila binges, to scary-sounding conditions she's encountered in her medical practice. But the show ultimately attributes her infertility to chance.

That's unique. Other media—and real-life people, in their casual conversations—subtly blame women for being unable to conceive. But *Grey's Anatomy* makes a point of blaming the randomness of the universe, not Meredith. Meredith cleverly calls out the unfairness of putting all the attention on women, when in reality, it takes two. She asks Derek how he'd feel if the doctor called his penis "angry or snide," like she called Meredith's uterus "hostile." Finally, the couple decides to put their infertility woes to rest, and they find joy in adopting their baby girl, Zola.[336]

For all its positive representations of infertility, though, *Grey's Anatomy* just couldn't leave Meredith and Derek as adoptive parents. Shortly after they bring Zola home, Meredith unexpectedly conceives.[337] It's like the show is saying: if you wait long enough, you too can overcome your infertility!

This is a running theme in a lot of media. Infertility isn't as taboo as it once was, and we see many shows, novels, and films trying to depict the grief of couples who want to have children, but can't. But what remains rare are representations of women who *stay* infertile, indefinitely. Everyone wants that happy ending, where the impossible happens. Take the film *The Odd Life of Timothy Green*. A couple who've just exhausted their fertility treatment options get to be "parents" when a 10-year-old boy magically emerges out of their garden, instantly knowing to call them Mom and Dad. This couple's pain is eased only with a literally magical solution to the "problem" of their infertility.[338] In this film and countless others, we don't see how couples grapple with and move past infertility; we only see them get the child they wanted all along.

Even more serious films don't leave us with couples yearning for parenthood. Thrillers and horror films have no problem showing us Bad Moms like Amelia and Eva; but leaving a barren couple childless would be too scary for viewers to handle. Psychological thriller *When the Bough Breaks* highlights how traumatizing infertility was for Laura and John: "I tried for so long to get pregnant," Laura says. "I had three miscarriages. It put the two of us through hell. You start to hate your own body." The couple decides to hire a surrogate, Ana, and Laura makes it her mission to make that baby hers—even when Ana extorts more money from them, seduces John, threatens to kill the baby, and then runs away with it. What's thrilling (and bizarre) about this film is that we never question Laura and John's motives. Overcoming infertility and getting the child they so desperately crave seem like perfectly viable reasons to make death threats and to *instruct* your husband to cheat on you. Baby mania, indeed.

We see this same absence of indefinitely infertile women in *Jane the Virgin*. We learn that Rafael and Petra's marriage began crumbling when Petra suffered miscarriage after miscarriage. Again though, her infertility "problem" is miraculously solved as soon as she artificially inseminates herself. Nine months later, Petra gives birth to perfect twins. We see it again in *Peaky Blinders*. While Grace and her husband seek treatment to help them conceive, she miraculously gets pregnant with Tommy's child. It's as though she was infertile because she was with the wrong man. And we see it yet *again* in cult-classic *Sex and the City*. Charlotte tries everything to get pregnant, from IFV to acupuncture. When she eventually remarries, they decide to adopt—only for Charlotte to show up with a baby bump later on down the line.

Viewers don't want to watch their favourite characters suffer. That's why plotlines involving infertility so often end with astonishing conceptions, adoptions, or surrogacy arrangements. Yet for many couples, permanent infertility is their reality. There are no little boys magically sprouting from the ground to fulfill their desire for children. How does it make these couples feel, to only see their struggle shown with an unrealistic fairy tale ending? Perhaps in the near future, we'll see plotlines where infertile couples can work through their grief and find happiness in ways other than becoming parents. But it hasn't happened yet.

The End of Life as She Knows It: Narratives of Teen Pregnancy

In the opening scene of *The Secret Life of the American Teenager*, a suburban mom reheats dinner for her teenage daughter, Amy. She puts pot roast in the microwave, while Amy, who's slipped away to the bathroom, carefully unwraps the pregnancy test she'd hidden in her tuba case. All the while, Amy's mom is going on about her intense band practices: "By the time you get home, you barely even have time to eat and do your homework, let alone have any fun! You're only young once; you should be having a little fun." We watch the microwave counting down to "0" while Amy takes the test. As the microwave flashes "END" across its display and blares its flatline-like alarm, Amy stares, horrified, at her positive test. She is about to pay the price for having the fun her mom chided her for missing out on. Life as she knows it is coming to an abrupt "END."

The Secret Life of the American Teenager both normalizes and questions behaviour like Amy's. On the one hand, it suggests all teenagers are getting themselves into these sorts of situations. They all have "secret lives" their parents don't know about. But on the other hand, the show constantly points out just how inappropriate Amy's pregnancy is. Right after that intro scene, for example, the show's theme song comes on: a bubble-gum pop melody that plays while colourful cartoon flowers and bumble bees scroll across the screen. And though her friends offer to go with her to see her doctor, they quickly realize they're already committed to yearbook meetings or ballet lessons—activities we're supposed to view as age-appropriate for these young-looking girls. We're meant to see Amy as a child who is way too young to be having the type of "fun" that got her into this predicament.

Then there are her parents' reactions: Amy's mother is totally flabbergasted, and her dad's furious with the baby's father. Both are also exasperated that Amy's entire school—and, more importantly, all their neighbours—have heard the news. We watch Amy try to deal with lots of practicalities—whether she should keep the baby, have an abortion, or arrange for adoption. But we also see Amy and her family try to manage the full-blown scandal her pregnancy causes.

Even the series' title is full of shock value. By using the singular pronoun—"*the* American Teenager"—the title implies that all American children are the same. They all lead "secret lives" that include taboo activities their parents would dread, including sex and pregnancies. *The Secret Life of the American Teenager* makes it seem like teens everywhere are living through these "adult" problems—even if adults don't know it.

Plenty of other shows take a similar, scare tactics approach to depicting teen pregnancy. Some shows think they can stop teen girls from getting pregnant—or even stop them from having sex—if they tell those girls they'll be desperately poor, hungry, and miserable if they have a baby. Look at MTV's *16 and Pregnant*: it's meant to be entertaining, first and foremost. But it was also designed to show viewers just how bad teen mothering can be, both for the mom and for her child. It shows plenty of new moms who are poor; who fight and break up with their boyfriends, even though they'd promised to stick around; and who can't finish school because they're exhausted. The idea is that, by showing young girls just how awful teen mothering is, fewer of them will risk pregnancy because they'll want to avoid this awful future at all costs.

But studies show that some girls, after watching *16 and Pregnant,* don't think teen mothering looks all that bad. Some of them say they can relate to the girls on the show; they think they have a lot in common. As a result, they ignore the negative effects of their pregnancy. So, the media's scary construction of teen pregnancy affects viewers in many, often unexpected, ways. We certainly can't rely on it to prevent teenagers from becoming unexpectedly pregnant.

Just look at all the other media floating around out there,

some of which even makes motherhood look glamorous for young women. "Keeping Up with the Kardashians," for example, profiles social media-influencer Kylie Jenner, who had her daughter when she was 20 years old. She's not a teenager anymore, but teenagers certainly idolize her. Jenner's picture-perfect life on Instagram makes it seem like motherhood is a breeze. But what you don't see on social media is all the extra support she has access to as a wealthy celebrity. The same goes for Sofia Vergara, an actor on the TV show *Modern Family*, who had her son at age 19. And for Grammy-winning singer Solange, who was 18 years old when she gave birth to her son. Many young girls look up to these celebrities as role models. That's not to say teenagers have babies because they're trying to imitate famous people. Rather, young celebrity moms might make teen parenthood look easier than it really would be for average girls.

Final Thoughts

"No time is the perfect time." That's a message we hear a lot in the media we've discussed this chapter. Look at *Jane the Virgin*. Getting accidentally artificially inseminated before you've launched your career or gotten married isn't ideal; it's ridiculous. But even though her careful plans are thrown out the window, Jane still crushes motherhood—and goes to grad school, lands a great job, and has no shortage of excitement in the romance department. The show implies that you don't need to tick everything off your To Do list before becoming a mom.

Grey's Anatomy is even more blunt. When Miranda's asked, "When's the best time to have children?" she responds: "Never … if you're waiting for the perfect time to have children, you're never going to have children."[339]

As much as I love Miranda, I disagree with her on this one. I think there *is* a perfect time to have kids: I tell you about it in the next chapter.

The problem isn't knowing what timing is perfect; we've got plenty of research to tell us that. The problem is *executing* that timing: actually *having* a baby at the optimal age and life stage. If the handful of examples we've discussed in this chapter are any indication, there are trillions of opinions floating around out there, pressuring people to live their lives in all sorts of conflicting ways. We're bombarded with these messages every day—and that's just from the media, never mind your friends, family, co-workers, and random strangers who feel entitled to give you their two cents. These beliefs sway our behaviour: they form our factor funnel, swirling our many other WiSK considerations around and shaping them into a final decision.

But these beliefs aren't always in our best interest. Think about the Baby Boomer belief that Millennials need to settle down and have kids ASAP. That timing won't work for the Millennial who can't find a job, nor for the Millennial who'll be in med school for the next five years. Or think about the conservative belief that abortion is not an option. You probably can't count the number of times I've said teen motherhood has disastrous consequences. Even though they're harmful, these beliefs still impact people's actions. Combined with the other factors in the WiSK funnel, beliefs play a role in making women have babies at far from perfect times.

So, again, our problem is execution: actually having a baby at the optimal time for your relationship, career, and personal goals. Until the beliefs I've been talking about change, many women will continue struggling to act on their WiSK decisions. The good news is, you've already taken the first step towards shaking the hold beliefs can have on you. Knowing that these beliefs exist, and questioning why we hold them, is the best way to set yourself up for independent decision making. And that's exactly what you've been doing for the past several dozen pages of this book.

CHAPTER SIX
The Best (and Worst) of Times

"It was the best of times, it was the worst of times …" In case you missed the reference, the title of this book is a nod to Charles Dickens' famous 1859 novel, *A Tale of Two Cities*. Anyone who made it through high-school English knows these lines from Dickens' book well. Though he wrote them to describe the French Revolution, they sum up the book in your hands perfectly. All the data, sociology, theorizing, cultural analysis—everything you've read in the preceding pages is meant to help us learn the best of times, and the worst of times, for a woman to have her first child.

Although less famous, the next few words in Dickens' book are equally important: "… it was the age of wisdom, it was the age of foolishness …" With these lines, Dickens was praising the big thinkers of the Scientific Revolution and the Enlightenment for their "wisdom." I'm talking about really smart people like Rene Descartes (the guy who coined the phrase "I think, therefore I am"), Denis Diderot (who had a hand in writing the first-ever encyclopedia), and Benjamin Franklin (the American Founding Father who discovered electricity and common sense). An age of wisdom, indeed. But as Dickens points out, it was also "the age of foolishness"—a time filled with oppression, hatred, and ultimately, years of suffering and bloodshed.

Fast forward to today, and Dickens' wise words still ring true. We live in an age of unparalleled wisdom. New discoveries and breakthroughs are being made faster than our blazing fast Wi-Fi can update us about them. And with 88 percent of Canadians online every day,[340] most people can easily find answers to the burning questions they have about basically anything. But, just as wise old Descartes, Diderot, and Franklin found themselves in a political mess that no amount of philosophizing could sort out, we too are living in an age of foolishness. Despite the unlimited information that's literally at our fingertips, too many people find themselves in less-than-ideal circumstances—circumstances that we have the power to prevent, by educating and empowering each other with the knowledge we already have.

Namely, we have a particular kind of wisdom within our reach. We know the answer to the big question we've posed in this book: when is the best time to have a child? We know the golden age—or life stage—that women should aim for. Yet this wisdom is constantly undermined by our own foolishness: by our refusal to do what research has shown is in women's best interests.

This doesn't mean women are foolish. It means that we, as a society, hold some foolish, outdated beliefs that make it hard for women to put this wisdom into practice. There are plenty of women who don't have the reproductive control that they should—that they have a *right* to. In many cases, it is the foolishness of harmful social systems—like patriarchy, sexism, and our love of shaming, to name a few—that is holding us back. Think about how many unplanned births we could prevent—and instead, how many women could have their children at the best of times—if we would stop clinging to these foolish beliefs:

- Teenagers should abstain from sex.
- Birth control is solely a woman's responsibility.
- Abortion is something women will regret for the rest of their lives.

In this chapter, I tell you the best (and worst) of times to have a child. Here, it's worth repeating something I said in the very first pages of this book: I'm not trying to tell you what to do. The research that follows is just that: research. And real life doesn't work like a science experiment. As we've seen in earlier chapters, there are plenty of reasons women might want or need to have children at times the research says are suboptimal. Whether it's values they learned growing up, their career dreams, their partners' own wishes, or a host of other variables, every woman's unique life experiences combine to shape her "best time" for a baby.

With that in mind, let's consider what the research suggests. It will take time and hard work for our society to become the supportive, unfoolish place that many women need it to be, in order to make use of this information. But that hard work begins by spreading the word about what we know, and about the changes that must be made in order to support couples in making good WiSK choices.

Questions you'll get answers to:

By "the best of times," I mean several different, but related, things. This isn't just a matter of the ticking biological clock. It's also a matter of the best time for a woman's career (if she has one), for her partnership (if she has one), and for her child (if she has one). So, I'll be answering the following questions in this final chapter:

▶ *At what age and life stage should a woman have a baby if:*
  ☑ *she also wants to pursue a career?*
  ☑ *she wants to give her partnership the best chances of lasting?*
  ☑ *she wants to set her child up for a healthy, happy life?*
  ☑ *she wants the best shot at a healthy, happy life for her-self?*
▶ *What about the worst of times? At what ages and life stages should women avoid pregnancy?*
▶ *How do the answers to these questions change for different women? For example, how are they different for women who were born rich, compared with those who were born poor? What about women with a lot of education compared with women with only a little? And how about single women compared with married women?*

Follow Goldilocks' example

Like most famous children's stories, *Goldilocks and the Three Bears* is pretty bizarre. Basically, a little girl, Goldilocks, wanders into a house inhabited by three human-like bears. There, she finds their breakfast laid out on the kitchen table and decides to help herself. But when she sits down at Papa Bear's place at the table, she finds the chair's too big and hard, the spoon's too heavy, and the porridge is too hot. So she gives Mama Bear's place a try, but the chair's too soft, and the porridge is cold. On her third and final try, Goldilocks finds her perfect porridge at Baby Bear's place: it's not too hot, it's not too cold—it's just right.

Goldilocks then decides to take a nap, so she heads upstairs and the same thing happens. Papa Bear's bed is way too big and hard for her liking, and Mama Bear's bed is too soft and squishy. But Baby Bear's bed is the perfect size, and not too hard or soft. It's just right.

The story ends when the bears return home and Goldilocks scampers away, unharmed. So there's no real moral to the story (except maybe not to trespass, or else angry bears will find you). But the story's mantra—the thing we all remember—is the very same message that women who want children should be empowered to follow through on. It's the take-home point of this chapter: women shouldn't have kids when they're too young, and they shouldn't have kids when they're too old. They should do it when the timing is just right.

That perfect timing—the sweet spot that will yield the best outcomes—is in your early thirties. By following Goldilocks' example, and setting themselves up just right, there will be positive results for everyone: for the mother's own happiness, for her relationship, for her career, and for her child's health and well-being.

How to Have It All

With celebrity Super Moms like Reese Witherspoon and Gwenyth Paltrow always on view—not to mention powerful fictional role models like Doctor Miranda Bailey—there's plenty of pressure on women to try to Have It All. But women who effortlessly juggle careers, marriages, and children are the exception, not the rule. Trying to do everything is undeniably stressful. So, if women want to prioritize their job over having children, or vice versa, they should be allowed to make that choice without being judged.

That said, most women today work, and most women are also mothers. We need to build a better system that lets them balance both sets of responsibilities. The solution—the way that women really can Have It All—has to do with *when* they have children. And when it comes to both women's careers and their partnerships, it pays to delay.

Disrupt Your Career at the Right Stage

Let's start with the relationship between age and career outcomes. It's safe to say that teen mothers have the worst time of it. They struggle to complete their education, which limits their job opportunities.[341] Many come to focus on how they'll put food on the table, rather than on how they can have a rewarding career.[342]

None of this should come as a surprise. We know to avoid pregnancy during our teens—but that's pretty much where common knowledge ends. The real question is: once you get out of those teen years, then what? Of all the years of adulthood to choose from, which are the best—the Goldilocks years—to become a mom if you also want a rewarding, successful career?

The answer is: your thirties. Women who have children in their twenties face larger wage penalties than those who delay into their thirties.[343] In other words, your financial future looks brighter if you start a family in your thirties than in (or before) your twenties.[344] Even delaying just a little goes a long way. One study found that delaying parenthood by one year increased a woman's salary by an average of 9 percent, work experience by 6 percent, and wages by 3 percent.[345]

For one, this is because women in their thirties will have finished school and made a solid start on their careers.[346] These more established workers will (rightly) feel more entitled to seek out promotions and raises. Women in their twenties, by contrast, will be either finishing school, or very green in the work world. A child could:

- interrupt their education;
- stop them from pursuing additional learning opportunities, like the post-grad certificates that go a long way in today's competitive labour market; and
- take them out of the job market right when a new opportunity opens up.[347]

One study traced the career paths of different "types" of women for 19 years.[348] The biggest group of women in this study—about 28 percent—were educated, had good earning potential, and gave birth in their twenties. These women took long maternity breaks—even longer than their government-paid leave. Eventually, they would start working again, and their earnings would gradually improve. But the long break caused permanent career damage. Their earning trajectory leveled off, compared with what it looked like before they went on maternity leave. Their earnings potential was stunted so much that it would never catch up with their initial potential, even after decades back at work.

Who's at risk for being one of these "late returners"—a woman who doesn't work for a long time after giving birth and stunts her earnings? Your chances *increase* until you reach age 30.[349] In other words, women's wages take a bigger hit the longer they stay on maternity leave.[350] And their chances of taking long periods of leave increase until they're thirty.

So when *should* you take maternity leave? Women who waited to get pregnant—and who got more education and better jobs first—earned more in the long run. So, women who go to school and get a foothold at work *before having children* are rewarded with higher paying careers.

Of course, things change depending on the type of work we're talking about.[351] A cashier will always have a different career trajectory than a lawyer. Cashiers need basic customer service skills, product knowledge, and some training to operate their till. They can learn these skills quickly, and they don't change much over time. Most cashiers' careers wouldn't be affected much by maternity leave. That's not true for lawyers. They constantly need to update their knowledge to keep up with rapidly changing laws, precedents, and professional practices. So, lawyers will take a bigger hit than cashiers for long maternity leaves.

That's why delaying is most important for highly educated women, and women with highly skilled jobs.[352] Maternity leave will always disrupt a woman's career. She'll always be "out of sight, out of mind" when it comes time for the boss to make decisions about promotions and raises. She'll also be missing out on valuable networking time. And, if her job is highly skilled and specialized, her skills could decay while she's away.[353] But these things are less likely to happen to women who have spent years building up their work experience. These women have a stable, well-paying job they can go back to after maternity leave. So, they will almost always be better off than women who leave before even getting a foothold.[354]

That said, even if you have an unskilled job, you're still better off delaying. That cashier might be able to go back to school if she decides to hold off on starting a family. Or she might be able to take on longer, more demanding shifts as a supervisor if she doesn't have to rush home to her children. Waiting until your thirties gives you time to lay the groundwork for a better-paying career.

Mind the Motherhood Wage Gap

In 2016, Kulp studied graduate students who were mothers. These women were always being pulled in two directions. They wanted to be Good Moms who put their child's needs first. But they also wanted to be model students who were devoted to their work. Despite their best efforts to juggle the two, their kids usually came out on top. These mothers had a hard time making connections. They were constantly being pulled away from networking opportunities like dinners, pub nights with professors, and conferences because they had to get home to their children. Because they hadn't made those connections, they weren't asked to co-author papers or guest lecture with their advisors. They were also less likely to be offered mentorships and to receive personalized career guidance. Some even had their commitment to their work questioned. Meanwhile, their childless peers were padding their CVs with all of these bonus opportunities. In the end, the mothers were at an obvious disadvantage when it came to competing for jobs or tenure.

Children always disrupt careers. Whether they do skilled or unskilled work, women's wages usually go down once they become mothers. This is called the motherhood wage gap: mothers earn less than women who don't have children.[355] And it gets worse the more children you have:

- Mothers with one child earn an average of 5 to 6 percent less than women who don't have children.
- Mothers with two children earn roughly 15 percent less than women who don't have children.[356]

The motherhood wage gap is essentially unavoidable. The most you can hope to do is soften the blow. To minimize the gap, your best bet is to—you guessed it—delay. Women who have children in their twenties are penalized more heavily than women who have children in their thirties.[357]

Stay Off the Mommy Track

We've all heard of the corporate ladder: the rungs you need to climb to get to the top. We'd all like to climb the most vertical ladder possible—one that takes us as high as possible, as fast as possible. But a lot of the time, it's men who get to climb up the corporate ladder. Women risk getting pushed on to the mommy track: a flattened career trajectory with fewer rungs that are further apart.[358]

When women have their first child, their employers tend to downgrade their responsibilities. They give the new mothers less important tasks. They also pass them over for training opportunities and new roles. Employers do this because they believe in Good Moms. They assume mothers will put their children first. In turn, employers assume mothers won't be able to meet tight deadlines, attend important meetings that fall outside of school hours, clock extra hours to ensure projects are completed, or do all the other things employees are expected to do to show they deserve a promotion. Some employers think they're being considerate, giving mothers the reduced responsibilities they must want. Others think they're protecting their business, ensuring things get done right and on time. Either way, employers give the important jobs to people they think can handle them—people who don't have kids competing for their time. But when they're put on the mommy track, women are put at a competitive disadvantage. They don't get opportunities to prove themselves, so they don't advance as far or as fast.[359]

Some women consider the mommy track a good choice:

a way to balance mothering with work.[360] But many women feel they're forced into it. They aren't asked if they want fewer responsibilities, or less demanding assignments; it's just assumed.[361]

It's called the "mommy track" because it's a problem that only women face. Compared to men and single women, mothers are less likely to be hired. They are also less likely to be seen as competent. Compared to men with the same qualifications, mothers also get paid less.[362]

Fathers don't face the same problems.[363] In fact, having children gives men a career boost: dads are more likely to be offered jobs than men without children. And those who already have jobs typically get raises after they become fathers.

That means men's wages tend to increase steadily with age, even as they marry and have children.[364] Women with the same qualifications see their wages increase with age too, but only until around age 27, on average. Then, we see them start to cut back on their working hours—and their wages decline. Their wages start to go up again once they get back into fulltime work, after their children are a little older. But by this point, mothers have less experience than men. They also have depreciated skills, compared to men. So, although their wages start going up again once they return to work, they never catch up with men's.

In the end, women seeking successful careers should give their employers no reason to doubt their dedication. They should not jump at the first chance to take maternity leave. Instead, career-minded women should wait to have children until they've built up a solid reputation, professional network, and significant work experience. In other words, women have to prove their abilities at work *before* they have children.

Of course, this isn't right or fair to women. But it is our reality. Employers shouldn't assume that children will "distract" women from their careers. But they often do assume just that. After all, child care falls disproportionately on mothers. Even those who work full time are usually responsible for the cooking, cleaning, diaper-changing, shopping, feeding, supervising, and the endless other duties that come along with having children. That's not fair, but it helps explain why employers are wary of demanding too much from mothers; they know their plates are already more than full.

Patiently Build Your Support System

This brings me to the second reason why it pays to delay. Women who are going to Have It All need the kind of strong, equal partnership that takes time to build. It's just not humanly possible to clock 80-hour workweeks while raising children all by yourself. Or at least, it's not possible to sustain that kind of life. Anyone who tries to keep it up for an extended period of time will either burn out or be a stressed, miserable mess—or both. The solution is finding a partner you can lean on and share the work with.

The key here is sharing. You don't just want *a* partner; you want a partner who treats you as their equal. You want a partner who's willing to split parenting with you 50/50. Being married to someone who expects you to do everything might be even more stressful than being a single parent.[365] At least single parents don't argue about who's failing to pull their weight.

So, being married doesn't guarantee happiness, just as being a single mom doesn't guarantee stress and misery.[366] But building an equal partnership can make parenthood less stressful by helping women share the burden. And you need time to build that kind of relationship.

Cue Goldilocks's return. There's a "perfect" age to get married—an age when you're not too young, and not too old. The sweet spot that's "just right" is between the ages of 28 and 32.[367] Couples who marry in these Goldilocks years have the best chances of staying together. Those who marry earlier or later are more likely to get divorced. The interesting thing is that these findings hold across different populations: race, education, religion, sexual history, and family background don't make a difference. No matter their demographic, people have the best shot at staying together if they get married between the ages of 28 and 32.

There are several reasons for the Goldilocks years of marriage. For one, people this age are more emotionally mature and financially stable than they were when they were younger. They've probably dated a few people and learned the difference between lust and love. They've had some experience with responsibility—with school, work, and independent living. So they're better prepared for the emotional responsibility of marriage. But, these 20- and 30-somethings are still young enough to be flexible. They're still growing and still open to their partners' needs. They're also unlikely to have ex-spouses or children from earlier unions who would compete for time, loyalty, and money.

There are also several reasons why these Goldilocks years bode well for women who want to Have It All. People who marry at these ages have the most stable, longest-lasting marriages. So that's a win on the relationship front. As we'll see below, it's also good for the kids' health and happiness—a second win for parents. Finally, delaying marriage until your late twenties or early thirties means women have time to focus on their career. They're not busy wedding planning when they should be studying for exams or job hunting. That's the final win for women's work life.

The last way couples can delay is after they get married. Marriages are more stable for couples who wait to have their first kid for a few years.[368] Those couples have time to build their life together, before it's interrupted with the stress of parenthood. So, reveling in your newlywed bliss is the best thing you can do for your marriage.

It's also the best thing women can do for their career. Taking a few years to settle into married life gives you time to figure out your relationship role and responsibilities. That is, it lets you figure out who's going to do what around the house. To repeat, more often than not, most of the cooking, cleaning, laundry, and other chores fall to women. If you want to have a rewarding career *and* children, you need to break that stereotype. Figure out an equal division of labour that works for you and your partner both. Take time to find an arrangement that lets each of you do what you're good at, and leaves each of you with time to relax and enjoy each other's company.

The Three Things that Help Children Reach Their Full Potential

In a survey of employers who were looking to hire, one manager reported: "The candidate opened his laptop and had his mother Skype in for the interview."[369] "One parent asked if she could do the interview for her child because he had somewhere else to be," said another. The sheer number of hiring managers who have been flabbergasted like this is hilarious. But this kind of ridiculous parenting behaviour is increasingly common. We all know at least one helicopter mom. These overbearing, protective mothers held their kid's hand through every second of their childhood. Why would they stop, now that those children are full-grown?

No one *wants* to be one of these annoying helicopter moms. People slip into the stereotype for all sorts of reasons. Most simply want the very best future possible for their child. But the reality is, some tried-and-true parenting tactics set children up for success. And helicopter parenting isn't one of them. All of those hiring managers—and jobless applicants—can back me up on this one.

Every parent wants to raise smart, sociable, successful children. To do that, parents need to do certain things with and for their children. These things fall into three categories:

1.   Parents need to provide basic necessities for their children—things like a safe home and food on the table. Some parents are better able to provide these things than others. That means children from poorer families have the cards stacked against them from the start. So, to give your children the best shot at a happy, healthy future, don't start a family until you're financially able to provide for one.

2.   Children turn out best when they're raised with some tried-and-true strategies. Like I said, helicopter parenting is really bad for children—but so is its opposite: neglect. The sweet spot is somewhere in between: a Goldilocks-approved middle ground known as the authoritative approach. I describe this approach—as well as some of the other, not so great approaches—below. Authoritative parenting makes children less likely to misbehave, act out, and get into trouble—not just as tod-

dlers, but as they grow into adults themselves.

3. Of course, there's more to parenting than getting your children to do as they're told. You want your children to do well in school and in life. For that to happen, children need to do activities that stimulate their cognitive, social, and sensory development. Parents are largely responsible for providing their children with these activities. So your child's future is in your hands.

Kids who get these three things—basic necessities, authoritative parenting, and stimulation—have the best chances of flourishing. How can you set yourself up to do all three? Delay motherhood until the Goldilocks years of your thirties.[370]

The first component is pretty obvious. Older, more educated, more financially stable parents are better able to provide food, shelter, and other necessities.[371] Women in their thirties have had time to finish school, get a good job, and grow up emotionally. So these women have the resources they need to satisfy these basic needs.[372] But the other two components are less obvious, so here's some more info about them.

Authoritative Parenting: Raising Well-Behaved Children

What exactly is authoritative parenting? In short, it's all about balance. It's about finding the mix of love and discipline that Goldilocks would say is "just right." Authoritative parents set limits for their children, but they're also warm and affectionate.[373] They make sure to provide fair, consistent discipline, and they explain to their children why the rules are the way they are. These parents listen to their children's needs, and they encourage them to be independent and opinionated, all while enforcing well-defined boundaries. So authoritative parents have high expectations for their children, but they're also nurturing and supportive. And they are usually rewarded for their diligent parenting with well-behaved children.

On the other hand, there's bad, authoritarian parenting. Authoritarian parents try to make their children follow the rules by harshly punishing them when they don't.[374] They don't bother explaining the rules to their kids. Those kids just know to expect a spanking if they don't do as they're told. Children usually have a hard time bonding with authoritarian parents. They struggle to feel emotionally close to the people who are harshly disciplining them. As a result, children raised by authoritarian parents are more likely to act out.[375] They reason they can behave however they want, so long as they don't get caught. By contrast, kids with authoritative parents have the information they need to make good decisions. So they're less likely to develop behavioural issues—whether at home, at school, or on the playground.

In short, you want to take an authoritative approach to parenting. It's good for you, because you won't become an overbearing helicopter mom. And it's also good for your children, who you'll be setting up to be well behaved, strong, and independent.

So how do you become an authoritative parent? The easiest way is to delay. Women who have children in their thirties are most likely to use this healthy parenting style. With a few extra years of life experience, these mothers are more mature, confident, established in their careers and relationships, and better able to keep their emotions in check.[376] In other words, they're less likely to snap when their toddler throws a temper tantrum, and less likely to retaliate with a spanking.

Younger mothers slip into authoritarian habits more easily. They're usually stressed, tight on money, and immature. That's a dangerous combination that can push them to use a heavy hand to discipline their children. One study found that teen mothers and even those in their early twenties used spankings, time-outs, and other harsh tactics more often than older mothers.[377] They intruded more on their child's privacy, were more controlling, and were more negative than older mothers. Other studies show that teen parents are more likely to take their anger out on their children.[378] And all of these authoritarian tactics make their children more likely to misbehave.

But we're not only talking about rowdy toddlers here. The effects of poor parenting shape a child's future. Once they're teens, youth born to teen mothers who use authoritarian tactics are at a higher risk for delinquency[379] and even gang membership.[380] Daughters of teen mothers are also more likely to become teen mothers themselves. That's another type of "delinquency" that puts their own children at risk for all of these dangers.[381]

There are many reasons that authoritarian parents tend to raise kids who act out. First, authoritarian parenting keeps parents and children emotionally distant. When children feel like they're alone, trapped in a harsh, punitive home, they often look for ways to escape their parents' reign. Drug and alcohol use, devious friends, and careless sex are all common—and dangerous—responses.[382]

Second, young, authoritarian mothers generally communicate poorly with their children.[383] Instead of explaining why their child needs to obey a curfew, an authoritarian mom would simply ground her daughter for getting home late. When children think rules are arbitrary, they don't feel their needs are being heard. Often, they start looking to other people to fulfill those needs—for example, to their boyfriends.

Once a child starts acting out, things usually just get worse. Mothers see their children slipping into bad behaviour, which makes them stressed. They feel they can't control their children, or that they're Bad Mothers because their discipline isn't working.[384] Then, they try to fix things by being even more strict and doling out harsher punishments. But that's what started the problem in the first place, so of course, it only makes things worse. And because young mothers are often more stressed to begin with—a product of their immaturity, and, often, their financial circumstances—these problems are biggest for teen mothers.[385]

On the other hand, authoritative parenting protects children from delinquency. When parents are involved in their children's lives, and enforce rules consistently, their children tend to have fewer friends who are "bad influences".[386] This is partly because children who live by their parents' rules don't have as many chances to get into trouble. For example, children who obey their parents' curfew aren't out late at night, wandering the streets or hanging out with the "wrong" crowd.

What's more, authoritative parents raise children who aren't as interested in that sort of thing. When parents forge an emotional bond with their children, showing that they're responsive to their needs and feelings, children are less likely to act out.[387] They're less likely to seek comfort in (or show off with) drugs and alcohol; less likely to distract themselves with dangerous activities and friends; and less likely to try to boost their self-esteem with sex.[388]

In short, good parenting makes for good kids. Poor parenting allows—and even promotes—children's misbehavior. And these tendencies toward risky behaviours follow people throughout their lives. People born to teen mothers are, as adults, more likely to lash out violently when frustrated.[389] They are even disproportionately likely to be imprisoned. Likely, that's because young mothers often struggle to provide supportive environments for their children, and to model good behaviours and values for them.

In sum, children turn out best if women have them when they're not too young, and not too old. You want to have them in the Goldilocks years of your thirties. Have them too early, and women risk becoming authoritarian parents who inadvertently promote behaviour problems,[390] including delinquency. But you don't want to have them too late, either. Once women pass 40, their children are less likely to enjoy the benefits of authoritative parenting—like good behaviour—and are instead more likely to develop some health issues, like obesity.[391] And as parents get older, they tend to have less energy for their children. They're less able or willing to play with their kids, and don't always have the patience to explain and enforce rules consistently. The Goldilocks-approved years are your thirties: becoming a mother beween the ages of 30 and 39 is "just right." Compared with women who become mothers in their twenties, these slightly older mothers tend to raise better-behaved children.[392] And, as we will see shortly, their kids tend to be smarter, and do better in school too.

Raising Smart, Sociable, Successful Children

Of course, there's more to parenting than raising obedient rule followers. Most mothers also want their children to make friends, do well in school, and eventually, hold a rewarding job. Their chances of succeeding in each of these areas depends on how well they're stimulated when they're young. And—you guessed it—older mothers have proven to stimulate their children more effectively than younger mothers.

Plenty of studies back that up. In one, researchers spent years interviewing mothers and videotaping them while they played with their children.[393] They saw that teen mothers were less supportive of their children and less responsive to their needs. They were even hostile towards their children when they were playing. The researchers wanted to see how those poor parenting strategies affected the kids. So, they compared three-year-olds born to teenagers with three-year-olds born to adult mothers. The kids of teen moms showed significantly worse cognitive and language abilities. The researchers concluded that the teen mothers' poor parenting strategies were holding their children back.

Another study compared five-year-old children born to mothers aged 18 or younger with five-year-olds born to mothers aged 25 to 34.[394] The kids of teen moms scored significantly lower on cognitive tests. In another study, the children of teen parents performed worse on literacy and math tests than children born to adult parents.[395] And in yet another study, children born to mothers under 20 years old were forty percent more likely to develop ADHD, compared to children of mothers aged 25 to 29.[396]

Here's why: teen mothers are unlikely to finish high school, let alone get a postsecondary education. That means they're also unlikely to hold down a stable, well-paying job that lets them support a family.[397] What's more, they're still children themselves. Yet, most have to live independently, without their own parents taking care of them. These four factors—education, income, social support, and immaturity—hold teen mothers back. Without these things, teen moms have slim chances of providing the kind of home that helps children learn and grow. These four factors also increase stress. Without the maturity, financial stability, and support that many older mothers have, parenthood feels all the more overwhelming.[398]

Here's some more detail on each of the four factors that make it hard for young mothers to raise smart, sociable, successful children:

1. Education

The younger the mom, the less likely she is to have finished school. And without schooling of their own, teen mothers probably aren't the best candidates to instill basic literacy or numerical skills in their children.

When women delay motherhood to get an education, their children have higher math and reading scores.[399] These more educated mothers spend more time with their children reading, drawing, talking, doing puzzles, and engaging in other activities that stimulate the brain and the senses.[400] On the other hand, teen mothers usually spend less time stimulating their children intellectually.[401] Their kids are more likely to watch lots of TV and to eat their meals alone.[402] As a result, these children typically lag behind those of adult mothers in motor, cognitive, and (as we saw earlier) behavioural skills.

2. Employment

Without much education, most teen mothers struggle to find stable, well-paying jobs. And without those jobs, they are less able to provide a stable home, and stimulating, educational activities for their children.[403] For example, they may not be able to afford the books, games, and toys that help children learn. Older mothers, on the other hand, are typically more financially stable. They can provide all of these things and more for their children.[404]

3. Social Circles

Children learn how to behave by watching and imitating the people around them. The people they're around most—their parents—have the greatest impact. This can be a problem for children of teen mothers. In a way, teen mothers are still children themselves; they're often immature and unfamiliar with adult interactions. The very fact that they're teen mothers suggests they are irresponsible and take life-changing risks.[405]

In general, teen mothers fail to conform to our values. Many got pregnant accidentally, much earlier than they wanted or intended. After getting pregnant, many do not get married, do not finish school, and do not move out of their parents' homes.[406] In short, they do not take the highway version of life that our society values. But now, they have children who are watching and imitating them. Those children learn to see their moms' behaviours and choices as normal. Teen mothers have not done as they were told, and often, neither will their children. At home, these children learn that it's okay to break the rules. So, not only do they break rules at home, they do so everywhere else too—at the mall, in restaurants, in daycare, and at school. Children of teen mothers are more likely to disobey their teachers. Their academic performance often suffers as a result.[407]

Teen mothers also tend to have small social circles. Some of their friends may disapprove of their choices. Others disappear because they're too busy with college applications and extra-curriculars. Usually, teen mothers don't have much in common with other mothers either. Older mothers judge them, assuming they're irresponsible or reckless. So, the children of adult mothers usually get play dates together, while those of teen mothers have fewer chances to interact.[408] And because their moms usually have few friends, these kids tend to have fewer positive role models.

4. Maturity

Even if they're wise beyond their years, teenaged mothers aren't fully mature, for biological reasons. That's because parts of the brain—namely, the prefrontal cortex—take a long time to develop. The prefrontal cortex is responsible for things like time management, paying attention, and concentrating on the task at hand. This part of the brain doesn't fully develop until we reach our twenties or thirties.[409]

As a result, teenagers aren't able to focus or prioritize as well as adults. These natural differences make older women better at parenting than teenagers.[410] It's not a stereotype; it's a biological reality. The younger a woman is, the less developmentally prepared she is for parenting. On average, adolescent mothers are much less supportive, sensitive, and affectionate towards children than adult mothers.[411]

There's an interesting experiment that showed this.[412] Researchers videotaped mothers as they tried to complete a questionnaire and supervise their children at the same time. Teen mothers had a hard time. They were less responsive to their child's needs, and less able to juggle the competing tasks. They were distracted by the questionnaire, which made them struggle to identify and address their infants' needs.

There's a lot more to parenting than letting your kid play while you fill out some paperwork. So let's unpack the implications of this experiment. It asks us to consider what happens when a teen mom is trying to watch her baby, cook dinner, and answer the phone between getting home from school and leaving for work. Answer: she's going to drop the ball on at least one of these things—and the experiment shows she doesn't necessarily have the skills to prioritize her baby over the other things competing for her attention. That matters because being responsive to your kids affects their development. Kids are more likely to meet their developmental milestones when they have responsive mothers.[413]

Some teen mothers may also be setting their children up for failure even before they're born. That's because teen mothers, on average, behave quite differently from adult mothers while they're pregnant. Women under the age of 20 are more likely to smoke, drink, and use drugs while pregnant.[414] That can harm a fetus's development. They are also less likely to receive prenatal care. Many teen girls don't even realize they're pregnant, or they may try to hide it from their parents. They can't get the medical attention or the information they need for a healthy pregnancy if they don't tell anyone they're pregnant. And inadequate prenatal care can lead to low birth weights and premature births that contribute to poor cognitive development.

For these four reasons—education, employment, social circles, and maturity—young mothers are more likely to raise children with poor cognitive and social development.[415] Their children don't develop literacy, numerical, or social skills as strongly or quickly as other children. As they age, these kids don't do as well in school. On the other hand, children whose mothers delayed childbearing enjoy important advantages. Just look at children born to mothers aged 30–34: they usually get a higher level of education than other children.[416]

Quality over Quantity

The problem isn't the amount of time mothers spend with their children. It's what mothers *do* with that time.[417] Do they leave their children in front of the TV for hours? Or do they read a book together? As we have seen, older mothers with more education and better jobs tend to choose healthier activities for their children.

So, it's a matter of quality over quantity. That's important for mothers—or mothers-to-be—who worry that work will get in the way of caring for their children. It's a common fear. Plenty of women are judged for "abandoning" their children to pursue their career. But remember: the simple act of delaying childbearing gives you much better odds of adopting authoritative, developmentally healthy parenting strategies. And that's true no matter how much time you spend at the office.

Nevertheless, people love taking sides in the so-called "mommy wars." They talk about working mothers versus stay-at-home mothers, and ask who's mothering better. Some would have us think that Good Moms are stay-at-home moms. These women, they say, make sacrifices so they can spend every minute focused on their children. So of course they raise the best-behaved, most successful kids. But that's not necessarily true. Childhood development has a lot more to do with the *ways* mothers interact with their children.[418]

Sociologists have sunk years into this debate. Study after study shows that there's no victor in the mommy wars. If you look at mothers who have similar levels of education and incomes, their kids usually have similar developmental outcomes. It doesn't make a difference if they work or stay home.[419]

One Canadian study stands out. In 2015, researchers Baker and Milligan set out to see if longer maternity leaves affected kids. Their study was spurred by a piece of Canadian legislation. Prior to 2000, mothers got 15 weeks of paid leave, plus an additional 10 weeks that could be split between new parents, for a total of 25 weeks. But for children born December 31, 2000 and onwards, that shared 10 weeks was expanded to 35 weeks. In effect, paid leave had just doubled, and mothers could take a total of 50 weeks paid leave. Some people loved this idea; they said it would give mothers more time to spend with their children during their first year of life. And that longer period would mean better cognitive development for children.

Baker and Milligan wanted to find out if that was true. It wasn't. As it turns out, the extra amount of leave didn't really change much. They looked at two-year-olds, comparing those whose mothers took the extra-long leave with those who did not. The kids were all similar in their motor and social skills development, temperament, and physical development.

Baker and Milligan took it a step further. They checked in on these children again when they were 4–5 years old—right before they started school. Again, all of the kids were pretty much the same in terms of their cognition and behaviour.

What does this mean for you? Well, if you choose to put your children in good-quality day care to go work, you shouldn't worry. Spending more time with your child won't boost their grades or turn them into social butterflies. Spending less time won't turn them into hermits or juvenile delinquents. A mother who works 50 hours a week, but reads her daughter a book before bed every night, is doing just fine. On the other hand, an unemployed high-school dropout who sits on the couch drinking all day will cause serious problems for her child's development—even though they spend more time together. Again, it's a matter of quality over quantity.

Bottom line: children of working mothers are not doomed to neglect. And children of stay-at-home mothers are not guaranteed the kind of attention they need to reach their full potential. Good mothering has more to do with your age and life stage. Teen mothers typically parent in less desirable ways than adult mothers. They are more likely to be authoritarian. In turn, these authoritarian practices tend to stunt their children's developmental, behavioural, and social progress. But women who become moms in the Goldilocks years of their early thirties are more likely to be authoritative. Thanks to these solid parenting practices, they set their kids up for success on all fronts.

Fostering Good Health

There's one last benefit to having children in the sweet spot of your early thirties: they're more likely to be healthy.

Children born to very young and very old mothers are at a greater risk for several health concerns.[420] When they grow up, these children tend to rate their own health more poorly, have higher-than-average rates of obesity, diabetes, and cancer, and run higher risks of mortality. Children of these very young and very old mothers are also more likely to develop mental health disorders later in life. On the other hand, women who became mothers when they were 30 to 39 are more likely to raise mentally healthy kids.[421]

Part of the reason for these differences is physiological. Both younger and older mothers are at a greater risk for low birth weight, pre-term birth, and other pregnancy complications. These can have long-term consequences for their children, including lower cognitive ability and poor health later in life.[422]

However, there are also sociological explanations. As we've discussed repeatedly, few teen mothers can afford nutritious food and healthy physical activities for their kids. But on the other end of the age spectrum, we see different problems. Older mothers are more likely to die while their children are still relatively young—at least, younger than women who were only in their twenties or thirties when they had children. As a result, children of older mothers may get less support and guidance over their lifetime. Without positive role models and a solid support system, these children may make poorer health decisions.[423] Losing a parent at a young age is also traumatizing. It can push youth and even adults to do unhealthy things—like drink too much, or use drugs—in their efforts to cope. And children of both much younger and much older mothers are predisposed to these behaviours to begin with; they're more likely to smoke, drink, and do other unhealthy things to cope with their stress.[424]

So, women who become mothers in the Goldilocks years of their thirties have the best chance of having healthy, well-behaved, smart, successful children. They're old enough to have the financial stability, maturity, and life experience they need to support children.[425] But they aren't so old that they're putting their children at risk for poor health. As Goldilocks would say, their timing is just right.

Making Motherhood the Joyful Experience We All Want It to Be

We all want answers to the questions asked in this book because we all want to be happy. Whatever you are planning—whether you want three children, a husband, and a white-picket fence, or you're planning to adopt, or you want to travel the world childfree—you're hoping to feel fulfilled. With that goal in mind, I looked at the research on happiness. I also looked at the research on unhappiness: on stress, dissatisfaction, and even depression. As you should be able to guess by now, if you're looking to have a family, the key to happiness is getting your timing right.

Several studies have asked how children affect our happiness. One compared young parents with childfree people of the same age. Unsurprisingly, the young parents were more stressed out.[426] The researchers then looked at stress, happiness, and mental well-being among older parents and non-parents. This older group reported very similar levels of well-being, whether they were parents or not. This suggests that slightly older adults are better able to handle the stresses of parenting than younger adults. In other words, you'll feel less overwhelmed if you delay having children until you're a bit older.

Other studies look at mothers specifically. To give yourself the best chances of being happy, you want to have kids in those Goldilocks years of your thirties. Your teens are too early: mothers under the age of 20 are more likely to experience depression.[427] But your forties are too late: women who give birth between the ages of 40 and 44 are also at a high risk of depression.[428] Your early thirties are just right: these women have the lowest risk for depression, and are usually happiest overall.[429]

So why are parents in their thirties happiest? Well, by the time they reach that age, they've usually hit plenty of milestones: finishing school, building their career, getting married, buying a house, and so on.[430] They're financially ready for parenthood, so they say they feel less stressed and better able to enjoy it.[431] But if they wait a little too long—until their forties—they'll endure criticism that takes some of the joy out of parenthood.[432] They'll be bombarded with questions about their fertility and whether it's safe for them to have children at their age.[433] And they will be reminded, as if they didn't know, that they don't have much time to spend with their children. So, even though they're excellent mother material in terms of their maturity and financial stability, older mothers can feel dissatisfied and unhappy.[434]

One study found these older mothers didn't necessarily *want* to wait. Many women want to have children earlier, in the Goldilocks years, but weren't ready. Some wished they'd found their partners earlier. Others didn't think they were financially stable enough. The women in this study felt these things were mostly out of their control. For example, how were they supposed to find their partners years before they did?

Nonetheless, they felt dissatisfied, often because of the values I discussed earlier. We tend to impose a "deadline" on mothers. It's an unspoken rule: a cut-off point after which childbearing is no longer acceptable. We know most people believe in this deadline. Look at the European Social Survey: it interviews people from 25 countries who are age 15 and up.[435] Over half (57.2 percent) say they think women's childbearing deadline is 40.

Older mothers can't ignore that. They know the *majority* of people think women shouldn't be having children after they turn forty. On some level, we all care what others think about us. This deadline pushes many women to have children earlier, while they are still in their thirties. That lets them avoid being seen as "too old" to become a mom. Women who delay their first pregnancy until their forties may find themselves the targets of gossip.

Final Thoughts

Things generally turn out better for women, and for the people they love, if they do things in a certain order, when they're a certain age. Here's the golden formula:

- Finish school.
- Start your career.
- Get married.
- Spend a few years enjoying newlywed life.
- Start trying to conceive when you're in your early thirties.

Of course, some people will need to put their own spin on this sequence. If your career plan involves a 10-year Ph.D., you'll need to get married before you've checked "finish school" off the list. But the basic principle of this golden formula still holds: many women will benefit from having a strong start on their career, and a solid foundation for their marriage, before they start thinking of having a baby. And women need to time these various phases in their lives so that they're ready to have their first child when they're in the Goldilocks years of their thirties.

Things aren't guaranteed to go south if you do things out of order. You're just more likely to come up against some serious obstacles. Here are just a few of the common consequences of doing things in the "wrong" order:

- Psychological distress
- Conflicting demands that cause stress
- Reduced satisfaction and happiness
- Conflict with your partner
- Stunted career growth

These bad things happen because our society is still structured to support the golden formula. If you deviate from it, you're going to get a lot of flak from your friends, family, and even random strangers. These people are going to judge you, they're going to think they know better, and they may even make you feel ashamed. These bad things also happen because our institutions—our schools, offices, government, and health-care system—are designed to fit the golden formula. Our society was made to help people experience life events at certain ages, in a certain order. So if you want the easiest path through life, all you have to do is follow the formula. Becoming a parent is really tough, but you can make it easier on yourself by being smart about your timing.

Of course, this doesn't mean you have to conform. If you know, without a shadow of a doubt, that you want to stay child-free, then you shouldn't let anyone make you feel badly for living your happiest life. Just know that you're going to come up against some opinionated, judge-y people who are going to try to drag you down. It takes a very strong, confident woman to keep those individuals from raining on her parade.

That's easier said than done. As you know from reading this book, there are powerful social forces pushing you to follow the golden formula. Forging your own path seems daunting, but it's a worthwhile undertaking that we should work harder to support. The only reason the golden formula produces the excellent outcomes I've outlined in this chapter is because we, as a society, continue to endorse it. We're the ones who insist that Good Moms must always put their children first—even (and maybe especially) above their careers. We're the ones who say it's weird when a man stays home with the children while his breadwinner wife's at work. We're the ones who push women onto the mommy track by leaving the brunt of childcare work to them. We're the ones who nag our own 20-something-year-old children about being single when it's in their best interests to delay anyway. And we're the ones who make women in their forties feel bad about having children so "late."

To reference wise old Charles Dickens again, we may live in an age of wisdom. But we're certainly messing it up for a lot of people, thanks to some of our foolish, outdated beliefs.

As a community, we have the power to change the way we look at parenting. Right now, the golden formula may be your best shot at leading a healthy, happy life and giving your children a good life—but it doesn't have to stay that way. By adjusting some of our traditional views, we can open up a world of possibilities that would give people the freedom to choose their own life course. Sure, it might never be safe for a 50-year-old woman to have a baby. But why can't she adopt without worrying that people will gossip or stare or think she's selfish for delaying, or ask if it's her grandchild? And on the other end of the age spectrum, will we continue to insist that abortion is a life-ruining mistake, but then let teens ruin their lives by forcing them to go through with unwanted pregnancies?

The research I've shown you throughout this book is meant to be empowering. It's intended to give women the information they need to make informed decisions about some of the most important parts of their lives. To put these pieces of wisdom to good use, we will have to let go of some of our more foolish ways. We will have to adopt more supportive, egalitarian views that help more women start their family at the best possible time.

Acknowledgements

In the summer of 2016, Dr. Lorne Tepperman and I had just published our second book together. We wanted to write another. An expert on family sociology (and master pin-pointer of the questions and concerns that seem to be on everyone's mind), Lorne brought up babies. People want to Have It All, he observed. But we haven't figured out how to make that happen—how to make sure that women who want a career don't have their ambitions derailed by diaper changing and day care drop offs. Lorne (rightly) figured that, as a 24-year-old childfree woman who'd just finished grad school and started her first "real" job, I'd have something to say on the topic.

We started digging through the mountains of research that would ultimately inform this book. It was a monumental task, made much more bearable thanks to a small army of talented undergraduate research assistants from the University of Toronto: Tamara Frooman, Marim Hashemi, Richard Kennedy, Nikhil Koduvath, Olivia Levy, Nasra Moumin, Rubitha Paramathas, Ashley Ramnaraine, Victoria Shi, and Sylvia Urbanik. Special thanks go to Zara Ahmad, for her editing skills and insights on decision-making models; Jill Foster, for her exceptional analyses of parenthood in the media; Emily Povse and Hannah Reaburn, for their impressive research abilities; and Madeleine De Welles, for her leadership as project manager.

I'm also deeply grateful to David Stover, my fantastic publisher, who championed this project from the start and was invaluable in whipping it into shape as it came to an end. Thank you, David, for your support, recommendations, and expertise.

But my biggest thanks go to Lorne, whose mentorship has opened so many doors for me over the last ten years. As someone who earns her living writing, you know it means a lot when I can't find words to express how much I've appreciated your wisdom, guidance, and encouragement in everything we've worked on together, and on this project in particular. This book wouldn't exist without you!

Notes

1. Rebecca Lindell and Leslie Young, "Meet the boomerang kids: 40% of young adults living with their parents," *Global News*, 2012, http://globalnews.ca/news/288198/meet-the-boomerang-kids-40-of-young-adults-living-with-their-parents/.
2. "Insights on Canadian Society Diversity of young adults living with their Parents," Statistics Canada, 2016, http://www.statcan.gc.ca/pub/75-006-x/2016001/article/14639-eng.htm.
3. Jeylan T. Mortimer and Phyllis Moen, *The Changing Social Construction of Age and the Life Course: Precarious Identity and Enactment of "Early" and "Encore" Stages of Adulthood* (Springer, Cham, 2016).
4. Martin Kohli, "The Institutionalization of the Life Course: Looking Back to Look Ahead," *Research in Human Development* 4.3 (2007): 253–271.
5. S.R. Hayford, K.N. Guzzo, and P.J. Smock, "The decoupling of marriage and parenthood? Trends in the timing of marital first births," *Journal of Marriage and Family* 76 (2014), 520-538.
6. Hande Inanc, "Unemployment and the timing of parenthood: Implications of partnership status and partner's employment," *Demographic Research* 32 (2015): 219.
7. Stacey Jean Bosick, "Crime and the Transition to Adulthood: A Person-Centered Analysis of At-Risk Boys Coming of Age in 1940s Boston, 1970s London, and 1990s Pittsburgh" (diss. Harvard University, 2009).
8. Mortimer and Moen.
9. Chris Gilleard and Paul Higgs, "Connecting Life Span Development with the Sociology of the Life Course: A New Direction," *Sociology* 50(2): 301-315.
10. Magda Nico, "Individualized Housing Careers in Early Adulthood: Conditions and Constraints in a Familistic Society," *Sociological Research Online* 15.1 (2010).
11. Michael X. Delli Carpini, "Baby Boomers," *The Forum* 12(3) (2014): 417-445.
12. Tomas Frejka and Tomas Sobotka, "Overview Chapter 1: Fertility in Europe: Diverse, delayed and below replacement," *Demographic Research* 19(3) (2008):15–45.
13. Dennis Hogan, "The Transition to Adulthood as a Career Contingency," *American Sociological Review* 45(2) (1980): 261–276.
14. Renee Richardson Ellis, *Interrelated Decisions? Timing of Transitions Out of Cohabitation in Relation to Other Life Course Events* (University of California, Irvine, 2010).
15. A. Metcalfe, M. Vekved, and S. Tough, "Educational attainment, perception of workplace support and its influence on timing of childbearing for Canadian women: A cross-sectional study," *Maternal and Child Health Journal,* 18(7) (2014): 1675-1682.
16. Elizabeth Schilling, "Non-linear careers: desirability and coping," *Equality, Diversity and Inclusion: An International Journal* 31(8) (2012): 725-740.

17. Magda Nico, "Variability in the the transitions to adulthood in Europe: a critical approach to de-standardization of the life course," *Journal of Youth Studies* 17(2) (2014): 166-182.

18. Krysia N. Mossakowski, "Unfulfilled expectations and symptoms of depression among young Adults," *Social Science and Medicine* 73 (2011): 729–736.

19. Jonathan F. Smith, Zlatko Skrbis, "A social inequality of motivation? The relationship between beliefs about academic success and young people's educational attainment," *British Educational Research Journal* 43(3) (2017): 441-465.

20. Mossakowski.

21. Heather M. Rackin and Christine A. Bachrach, "Assessing the Predictive Value of Fertility Expectations Through a Cognitive–Social Model," *Population Research and Policy Review* 35(4) (2016): 527-551.

22. Paul E. Panek, Sara Staats, and Amanda Hiles, "College Students' Perceptions of Job Demands, Recommended Retirement Ages, and Age of Optimal Performance in Selected Occupations," *International Journal of Aging and Human Development* 62.2 (2006): 87–115.

23. Nico, *Variability in the the transitions to adulthood in Europe.*

24. Janel E. Benson and Glen H. Elder Jr., "Young Adult Identities and Their Pathways: A Developmental and Life Course Model," *American Psychological Association* 47.6 (2011): 1646-1657.

25. Christie Sennott and Stefanie Mollborn, "College-bound teens' decisions about the transition to sex: Negotiating competing norms," *Advances in Life Course Research* 16(2) (2011): 83-97.

26. Ellis.

27. Ellis.

28. Hayford, Guzzo, and Smock.

29. Anne H. Gauthier, "Family Policies in Industrialized Countries: Is There Convergence?" *Population* 57(3) (2002): 447–474.

30. A. Trimarci and J. Van Bevel, "Education and the transition into fatherhood: The role of selection into union," *Demography* 54 (2017): 119-144.

31. Juliet Stone et al., "The changing determinants of UK young adults´ living arrangements," *Demographic Research* 25 (2011): 629–660.

32. Ellis.

33. Jeffrey Jensen Arnett, "Emerging Adulthood: What Is It, and What Is It Good For?," *Child Development Perspectives* 1(2) (2007): 68-73.

34. Rachel Arocho and Claire M. Kamp Dush, "Like mother, like child: Offspring marital timing desires and maternal marriage timing and stability," *Journal of Family Psychology* 31(3) (2017): 261-272.

35. Arocho and Dush.

36. Patrick Heuveline and Jeffrey M. Timberlake, "The role of cohabitation in family formation: The United States in Comparative Perspective," *Journal of Marriage and Family* 66(5) (2004): 1214-1230.

37. Hayford, Guzzo, and Smock.

38. "Custody, Access and Child Support: Findings from The National Longitudinal Survey of Children and Youth," Government of Canada, Department of Justice, Electronic Communications, accessed February 1, 2018, http://www.justice.gc.ca/eng/rp-pr/fl-lf/famil/anlsc-elnej/p2_01.html.

39. Ellis.

40. Kieron Barclay and Mikko Myrskyla, "Advanced Maternal Age and Offspring Outcomes: Reproductive Aging and Counterbalancing Period Trends," *Population and Development Review* 42(1) (2016): 69-94.
41. Amanda Black et al., "Chapter 1: Contraception in Canada," *Journal of obstetrics and gynaecology Canada* 37.10 (2015): S5–S12.
42. Arocho and Dush.
43. Christin Hilgeman and Carter T. Butts, "Women's employment and fertility: A welfare regime paradox," *Social Science Research* 38(1) (2009): 103-117.
44. Aliaksandr Amialchuk, "The effect of husband's job displacement on the timing and spacing of births in the United States," *Contemporary Economic Policy* 31(1) (2013): 73-93.
45. Ibid.
46. Carola Eriksson et al., "Reflections on fertility and postponed parenthood—interviews with highly educated women and men without children in Sweden," *Upsala Journal of Medical Sciences* 118(2) (2013): 122-129.
47. Dirgha Ghimire, "Wives' and Husbands' Nonfamily Experiences and First-Birth Timing," *International Journal of Sociology* 45(1) (2015): 4–23.
48. Hilgeman and Butts.
49. Melinda Mills et al., "Why do people postpone parenthood? Reasons and social policy incentives," *Human Reproduction Update* 17(6) (2011): 848–860.
50. Metcalfe, Vekved, and Tough.
51. Ghimire.
52. R. Thompson and C. Lee, "Sooner or later? Young Australian men's perspectives on timing of parenthood," *Journal of Health Psychology* 16(5) (2011): 807–818.
53. Ghimire.
54. Jennie E. Brand and Dwight Davis, "The Impact of College Education on Fertility: Evidence for Heterogeneous Effects," *Demography* 48 (2011): 863–887.
55. Metcalfe, Vekved, and Tough.
56. Mills et al.
57. Hilgeman and Butts.
58. Jennifer C. Day, "Age at first birth and the pacing of subsequent births: A cohort Analysis" (Ph.D., The American University, 1994).
59. Amialchuk.
60. Benoit Laplante, "The well-being of families in Canada's future," *Canadian Studies in Population,* 1.2 (2018): 24–32.
61. Hilgeman and Butts.
62. Henriette Engelhardt and Alexia Prskawetz, "On the Changing Correlation Between Fertility and Female Employment over Space and Time," *European Journal of Population* 20(1) (2004): 35-62.
63. Amialchuk.
64. Massimiliano Bratti and Laura Cavalli, "Delayed First Birth and New Mothers' Labor Market Outcomes: Evidence from Biological Fertility Shocks," *European Journal of Population* 30(1) (2014): 35–63.
65. Engelhardt and Prskawetz.
66. A. Adersa, "Changing fertility rates in developed countries. The impact of labor market Institutions," *Journal of Population Economics* 17 (2004):17–43.

67. Adersa.
68. Adersa.
69. Adersa.
70. Arocho and Dush.
71. T. Sobotka, V. Skirbekk, D. Philipov, "Economic recession and fertility in the developed world," *Population and Development Review, 37*(2) (2011), 267-306.
72. Amialchuk.
73. Frejka and Sobotka.
74. Hilgeman and Butts.
75. M. Shannon and D. Grierson, "Mandatory retirement and older worker employment," *Canadian Journal of Economics* 37(3) (2004): 528-551.
76. Suh-Ruu Ou and Arthur J. Reynolds, "Timing of First Childbirth and Young Women's Postsecondary Education in an Inner-City Minority Cohort," *Urban Education* 48(2) (2013): 289-313.
77. Arocho and Kent.
78. Marisa Matias and Anne Marie Fontaine, "Intentions to Have a Child: A Couple-Based Process," *Family Relations Interdisciplinary Journal of Applied Family Science* 66(2) (2017): 231-243.
79. T. Burns and E. Roszkowska, "Rational Choice Theory: Toward a psychological, social, and material contextualization of human choice behavior," *Theoretical Economics Letters, 6*(2) (2016), 195-207.
80. S. Brown, ""They think it's all up to the girls": Gender, risk and responsibility for contraception," *Culture, Health & Sexuality,* 17(3) (2015): 312–325.
81. X. L. Ang, "The effects of cash transfer fertility incentives and parental leave benefits on fertility and labor supply: Evidence from two natural experiments," *Journal of Family and Economic Issues,* 36(2) (2015), 263-288.
82. R. Beaujot, C. J. Du, and Z. Ravanera, "Family policies in Quebec and the rest of Canada: Implications for fertility, child-care, women's paid work, and child development indicators," *Canadian Public Policy,* 39(2) (2013), 221-240.
83. Hilgeman and Butts.
84. Ang.
85. A. Luci-Greulich and O. Thevenon, "The impact of family policies on fertility trends in developed countries. European Journal of Population," *Revue Européenne De Démographie* 29(4) (2013), 387-416.
86. Anne H. Gauthier, "The impact of family policies on fertility in industrialized countries: a review of the literature," *Population Research and Policy Review* 26(3) (2007): 323-346.
87. A. Kemnitz and M. Thum, "Gender power, fertility, and family Policy," *The Scandinavian Journal of Economics,* 117(1) (2015), 220-247.
88. Beaujot, Du, and Ravanera.
89. Amialchuk.
90. Gauthier.
91. Luci-Greulich and Thevenon.
92. Kemitz and Thum.
93. Engelhardt and Prskawetz.
94. Arnstein Aassve and Trude Lappegard, "Cash-Benefit Policy and Childbearing Decisions in Norway," *Marriage and Family Review* 46(3) (2010): 149-169.

95. Melissa A. Milkie, Kei M. Nomaguchi, Kathleen E. Denny, "Does the Amount of Time Mothers Spend With Children or Adolescents Matter?" *Journal of Marriage and Family* 77(2) (2015): 355-372.
96. Keminitz and Thum.
97. Aassve and Lappegard.
98. Margaret L. De Wit, "Educational Attainment and Timing of Childbearing Among Recent Cohorts of Canadian Women," (Ph.D., The University of Western Ontario, 1993).
99. Rackin and Bachrach.
100. R. Jones and L. Frohwirth, "More than poverty: disruptive events among women having abortions in the USA," *The Journal of Family Planning and Reproductive Health Care* 39(1) (2013): 36.
101. Arocho and Dush.
102. Milkie, Nomaguchi, and Denny.
103. Ellis.
104. Kevin Shafer, Todd M. Jensen, and Erin K. Holmes, "Divorce Stress, Stepfamily Stress, and Depression among Emerging Adult Stepchildren," *Journal of Child and Family Studies* 26(3) (2017): 851-862.
105. Elizabeth Wall-Wieler, et al., "Teenage pregnancy: The impact of maternal adolescent childbearing and older sister's teenage pregnancy on a younger sister," *BMC Pregnancy and Childbirth* 16(1) (2016): 120–132.
106. Perrier (2013).
107. Hayford, Guzzo, and Smock.
108. Arocho and Dush.
109. Nitzan Peri-Rotem, "Religion and Fertility in Western Europe: Trends Across Cohorts in Britain, France and the Netherlands," *European Journal of Population* 32(2) (2016): 231-265.
110. Jeremy E. Uecker and Jonathan P. Hill, "Religious Schools, Home Schools, and the Timing of First Marriage and First Birth," *Review of Religious Research* 56(2) (2014): 189-218.
111. Uecker and Hill.
112. Peri-Rotem.
113. Peri-Rotem.
114. Deborah A. Widdowson et al., "Why go to school? Student, parent and teacher beliefs about the purposes of schooling," *Asia Pacific Journal of Education* 35(4) (2015): 471-484.
115. Hayford, Guzzo, and Smock.
116. Hayford, Guzzo and Smock.
117. Ellis.
118. Mills et al.
119. Ghimire.
120. Ellis.
121. Mortimer et al.
122. Jacob Dunbar. (2014). Re: *We Need to Talk about Kevin (2011) Trailer* [Video file]. Retrieved from https://www.youtube.com/watch?v=ZLR-gAe2jLaw.
123. Miller McPherson et al., "Birds of a Feather: Homophily in Social Networks," *Annual Review of Sociology* 27(2001): 415-444.
124. Dunbar.
125. Jones and Frohwirth.
126. Jones and Frohwirth.

127. M. Soderberg et al., "Women's attitudes towards fertility and childbearing: A study based on a national sample of Swedish women validating the Attitudes to Fertility and Childbearing Scale (AFCS)," *Sexual & Reproductive Healthcare* (2015): 1–5.
128. Ann Berrington, "Perpetual postponers? Women's, men's and couple's fertility intentions and subsequent fertility behaviour," *Population Trends 117* (2004), 9–19.
129. Berrington.
130. David Voas, "Conflicting Preferences: A Reason Fertility Tends to Be Too High or Too Low," *Population and Development Review* 29(4) (2003): 627–646.
131. Maria Iacovou and Lara Patricio Tavares, "Yearning, Learning, and Conceding: Reasons Men and Women Change Their Childbearing Intentions," *Population and Development Review* 37(1) (2011): 89-123.
132. Maria Rita Testa, Laura Cavalli, and Alessandra, "The Effect of Couple Disagreement about Child-Timing Intentions: A Parity-Specific Approach," *Population and Development Review* 40(1) (2014): 31-53.
133. Voas.
134. Berrington.
135. Voas.
136. Elyse Jennings, "The Influence of Wives' and Husbands' Fertility Preferences on Progression to Higher Parity Pregnancies in Nepal," *Population Association of America* (2013).
137. Aassve and Lappegard.
138. Aassve and Lappegard.
139. Milkie, Nomaguchi, and Denny.
140. Vikesh Amin and Jere R. Behrman, "Do more-schooled women have fewer children and delay childbearing? Evidence from a sample of US twins," *Journal of Population Economics* 27(1) (2014): 1-31.
141. Karel Neels et al., "Rising Educational Participation and the Trend to Later Childbearing," *Population and Development Review* 43(4) (2017): 667-693.
142. Ghimire.
143. Tomas Sobotka and Eva Beaujouan, "Two Is Best? The Persistence of a Two-Child Family Ideal in Europe," *Population and Development Review* 40(3) (2014): 391-419.
144. Iacovou and Tavares.
145. Iacovou and Tavares.
146. Ghimire.
147. Gauthier.
148. Gauthier.
149. Amialchuk.
150. Mary Stewart and Kirsten Black, "Choosing a combined oral contraceptive pill. *Australian Prescriber* 38(1) (2015): 6–11.
151. L. Bassett, "Donald Trump taps anti-contraceptive activist to oversee family planning Program," *The Huffington Post*, 2017, http://www.huffingtonpost.com/entry/teresa-manning-contraception-hhsu-s5907582ae4b05c397680d921.
152. C. Davies, "Poland's abortion ban proposal near collapse after mass protests. *The Guardian*, 2016, https://www.theguardian.com/world/2016/oct/05/polish-government-performs-u-turn-on-total-abortion-ban.

153. "Ontario sex-ed protest 'unlike anything I've ever experienced,' principal says," *CBC News*, October 1, 2015, http://www.cbc.ca/news/canada/toronto/ontario-sex-ed-protest-1.3251799.

154. The Canadian Press, "Parents against sex education to protest at Queen's Park," *City News*, 2016, http://www.citynews.ca/2016/09/21/parents-against-sex-education-to-protest-at-queens-park/.

155. Sarah R. Hayford and Karen Benjamin Guzzo, "Fifty Years of Unintended Births: Education Gradients in Unintended Fertility in the US, 1960-2013," *Population and Development Review* 42(2) (2016): 313-341.

156. Tomas Sobotka and Ava Beaujouan, "Late motherhood in low-fertility countries: Reproductive intentions, trends and consequences," *Preventing Age Related Fertility Loss* (2017).

157. A. Metcalfe et al., "Exploring the relationship between socioeconomic factors, method of contraception and unintended pregnancy. *Reproductive Health* 13(28) (2016): 1–8.

158. "Contraception," Centers for Disease Control and Prevention, 2017, https://www.cdc.gov/reproductivehealth/contraception/.

159. Black et al.

160. Centers for Disease Control and Prevention, *Contraception*.

161. Z. McKnight, "Don't worry, you can still get an IUD in Canada—if you have insurance," *Toronto Star*, 2017, https://www.thestar.com/life/2017/01/31/dont-worry-you-can-still-get-an-iud-in-canada-if-you-have-insurance.html.

162. Black et al.

163. Stewart and Black.

164. Stewart and Black.

165. A. Norton, "Women overestimate effectiveness of the pill, condoms," *Toronto Star*, 2012, https://www.thestar.com/life/health_wellness/2012/04/27/women_overestimate_effectiveness_of_the_pill_condoms.html.http://planb.ca.

166. J. J. Frost et al., "Young adults' contraceptive knowledge, norms and attitudes: Associations with risk of unintended pregnancy, *Perspectives on Sexual and Reproductive Health*, 44(2) (2012): 107–116.

167. Cleland et al. (2014).

168. Norton.

169. Philip DeCicca and Harry Krashinsky, "Does Education Reduce Teen Fertility? Evidence from Compulsory Schooling Laws," *The National Bureau of Economic Research* (2015), Working Paper No. 21594.

170. J.A. Behrman, "Does schooling affect women's desired fertility? Evidence from Malawi, Uganda, and Ethiopia," *Demography*, 52 (2015): 787–809.

171. Metcalfe et al.

172. Black et al.

173. "Learn About OHIP+," *Ontario*, <https://www.ontario.ca/page/learn-about-ohip-plus>.

174. McKnight.

175. McKnight.

176. A. Dennis and D. Grossman, "Barriers to contraception and interest in over-the-counter access among low-income women: A qualitative study," *Perspectives on Sexual and Reproductive Health* 44(2) (2012): 84–91.

177. Jenifer E. Allsworth et al, "Differences in contraceptive discontinuation among black and white women: Evidence from the Contraceptive CHOICE project," *Journal of Women's Health* 27(5) (2018): 599–606.
178. M. Wilde and S. Danielsen, "Fewer and better children: Race, class, religion, and birth control reform in America," *American Journal of Sociology* 119(6) (2014): 1710–1760.
179. Wilde and Danielsen.
180. Dennis and Grossman.
181. Norton.
182. L. Tousignant, "'Stealthing' is the newest dangerous sex trend," *New York Post,* 2017, http://nypost.com/2017/04/24/stealthing-is-the-newest-dangerous-sex-trend/.
183. J. N. Bergmann and J.K. Stockman, "How does intimate partner violence affect condom and oral contraceptive use in the United States? *Contraception* 91(6) (2015): 438–455.
184. K. Grace and J. Anderson, "Reproductive coercion: A systemic review," *Violence and Abuse* (2016).
185. Grace and Anderson.
186. Grace and Anderson.
187. Wildsmith et al. (2015).
188. Brown.
189. Brown.
190. Brown.
191. Maclaurin-Jones et al. (2016).
192. "Chapter 3: Emergency Contraception," *Journal of Obstetrics and Gynaecology Canada* 37(10) (2015): S20–S28.
193. "Morning-After Pill (Emergency Contraception)," Planned Parenthood, 2017, https://www.plannedparenthood.org/learn/morning-after-pill-emergency-contraception.
194. See planb.ca.
195. Sophia Yen et al., "Emergency contraception pill awareness and knowledge in uninsured adolescents: High rates of misconceptions concerning indications for use, side effects, and access," *Journal of Pediatric and Adolescent Gynecology* 28(5) (2015): 337–42.
196. Metcalfe et al.
197. A. Clack and P. Lledo-Weber, "Ensuring that women have access to safe abortion is "pro life," *BMJ* (2012).
198. "Abortion Services Now Available in the Province of Prince Edward Island," Abortion Rights Network, 2017, http://www.abortionrightspei.com.
199. Clack and Lledo-Weber.
200. S. Herold et al., "Women's private conversations about abortion: A qualitative study. *Women & Health,* 55(8) (2015): 943–959.
201. Paul Saurette and Kelly Godron, "The Changing Voice of the Anti-Abortion Movement: The Rise of Pro-Woman Rhetoric in Canada and the United States, *Toronto: University of Toronto Press* (2016).
202. Saurette and Gordon.
203. Clack and Lledo-Weber.
204. Black et al.
205. F. Hanschmidt et al. "Abortion stigma: A systemic review, *Perspectives on Sexual and Reproductive Health* 48(4) (2016): 169–177.
206. Metcalfe et al.

207. E. Wiebe, "Contraceptive practices and attitudes among immigrant and nonimmigrant women in Canada," *Canadian Family Physician* 59(10) (2013): 451–455.
208. Saurette and Gordon.
209. "About Us," Silent No More Awareness, 2018, http://www.silentnomoreawareness.org/about-us/index.aspx.
210. R. Graham, "The Myth of Abortion Regret," *Slate*, 2016, http://www.slate.com/articles/double_x/doublex/2016/10/the_myth_of_abortion_regret.html.
211. Corinne H. Rocca et al., "Decision rightness and emotional responses to abortion in the United States: A longitudinal study, *PLOS One*, 2015, http://journals.plos.org/plosone/article?id=10.1371/journal.pone.0128832#sec014.
212. Graham.
213. Ralph et al. (2017).
214. L.J. Ralph, et al., "Measuring decisional certainty among women seeking abortion," *Contraception* 95 (2017): 269–278.
215. Herold et al.
216. Rocca et al.
217. K. Kimport et al., "Addressing the silence in the noise: How abortion support talklines meet some women's needs for non-political discussion of their experiences," *Women & Health* 52(1) (2012): 88–100.
218. Herold et al.
219. D. Schmitz, "Terminating pregnancy after prenatal diagnosis–with a little help of professional ethics?," *Journal of Medical Ethics* 38 (2012): 399–402.
220. E Hurford et al., "The decision to continue a pregnancy affected by Down syndrome: Timing of decision and satisfaction with receiving a prenatal diagnosis. *Journal of Genetic Counseling*, 22(5) (2013): 587–593.
221. Susana Nuccetelli, "Abortion for fetal defects: Two current arguments." *Medicine, Health Care and Philosophy* 20 (3) (2017): 447–450.
222. E. F. France et al., "Imagined futures: How experiential knowledge of disability affects parents' decision making about fetal abnormality. *Health Expectations* 15(2) (2012): 139–156.
223. Brown.
224. Jessica Silk and Diana Romero, "The role of parents and families in teen pregnancy prevention: An analysis of programs and policies," *Journal of Family Issues* 35 (10) (2014): 1339–1362.
225. J.M. Grossman et al., "Protective effects of middle school comprehensive sex education with family involvement. *Journal of School Health*, 84(11) (2014): 739–747.
226. Kathrin F. Stranger-Hall and David W. Hall, "Abstinence-only education and teen pregnancy rates: Why we need comprehensive sex education in the U.S," *PLoS ONE* 6(10) (2011): e24658–e24658.
227 "Initial Report on Public Health: Teen Pregnancy," Ministry of Health and Long-Term Care, 2017, http://www.health.gov.on.ca/en/public/publications/pubhealth/init_report/tp.html.
228. Silk and Romero.
229. Wall-Wieler et al.
230. Metcalfe et al.
231. Silk and Romero.

232. J. Cleland et al., "Unmet need for contraception: Issues and challenges, *Studies in Family Planning* 45(2) (2014): 105–122.
233. Silk and Romero.
234. Stranger-Hall and Hall.
235. Silk and Romero.
236. V. Millner et al., "Parents' beliefs regarding sex education for their children in Southern Alabama public schools," *Sex Res Soc Policy* 12 (2015): 101–109.
237. Ellis.
238. R.H. Farr et al., "Microaggressions, feelings of difference, and resilience among adopted children with sexual minority parents. *Journal of Youth and Adolescence,* 45(1) (2016): 85–104.
239. D. Lupton, "A love/hate relationship: The ideals and experiences of first-time mothers," *Journal of Sociology* 36(1) (2000): 50–63.
240. J. Maher and L. Saugeres, "To be or not to be a mother?: Women negotiating cultural representations of mothering," *Journal of Sociology* 43(1) (2007): 5–21.
241. B. Fox, "The formative years: How parenthood creates gender, *The Canadian Review of Sociology and Anthropology* 38(4) (2001): 373–390.
242. C. Malacrida and T. Boulton, "Women's perceptions of childbirth "choices": Competing discourses of motherhood, sexuality, and selflessness," *Gender and Society* 26(5) (2012): 748–772.
243. Lupton.
244. Maher and Saugeres.
245. K. Gentile, "Reply to commentaries: "What about the baby? The new cult of domesticity and media images of pregnancy," *Studies in Gender and Sexuality,* 12(1) (2011), 72–77.
246. Fox.
247. A. Patel, "Mothers talk candidly about postpartum depression: "You're not alone," *Global News,* 2017, http://globalnews.ca/news/3417263/postpartum-depression-signs/.
248. "Postpartum depression more common in urban areas," *CBC,* 2013, http://www.cbc.ca/news/health/postpartum-depression-more-common-in-urban-areas-1.1409996.
249. L. Held and A. Rutherford, "Can't a mother sing the blues? Postpartum depression and the construction of motherhood in late 20th-century America," *History of Psychology* 15(2) (2012): 107-123.
250. Held and Rutherford.
251. Patel.
252. Held and Rutherford.
253. P. Tomasi, "A massive postpartum depression study has just opened in Canada," *Huffington Post,* 2017, http://www.huffingtonpost.ca/2017/04/27/postpartum-depression-study_n_16272462.html.
254. Patel.
255. Gentile.
256. Malacrida and Boulton.
257. Malacrida and Boulton.
258. Malacrida and Boulton.
259. Lupton.
260. Maher and Saugeres.
261. Gentile.

262. D. Saunders, "I really regret it. I really regret having children," *The Globe and Mail*, 2007, https://www.theglobeandmail.com/life/parenting/mothers-day/i-really-regret-it-i-really-regret-having-children/article1200668/?page=all.
263. Gentile.
264. O. Khazan, "How people decide whether to have children," *The Atlantic*, May 22, 2017, https://www.theatlantic.com/health/archive/2017/05/how-people-decide-whether-to-have-children/527520/.
265. A. Bays, "Perceptions, emotions, and behaviors toward women based on parental status," *Sex Roles* 76 (2017): 138–155.
266. Pearl Dykstra and Gunhild Hagestad, "Roads less taken," *Journal of Family Issues* 28(10) (2007): 1275-310.
267. Frederick Wyatt, "A clinical view of parenthood," *Bulletin of the Menninger Clinic* 35.3 (1971): 167.
268. Dykstra and Hagestad.
269. Maher and Saugeres.
270. Bays.
271. Bays.
272. Maher and Saugeres.
273. Gentile.
274. Thomas Hansen, "Parenthood and happiness: A review of folk theories versus empirical Evidence," *Social Indicators Research* 108.1 (2012): 29–64.
275. Hansen.
276. Soderberg et al.
277. Khazan.
278. L. Ibisomi and N.N. Mudege, "Childlessness in Nigeria: perceptions and acceptability," *Culture, Health & Sexuality* 16(1) (2014): 61–75.
279. Maher and Saugeres.
280. Hansen.
281. Maher and Saugeres.
282. Gentile.
283. J. Wakefield et al., "The nation and the family: The impact of national identification and perceived importance of family values on homophobic attitudes in Lithuania and Scotland," *Sex Roles* 75(9–10) (2016): 448–458.
284. B. Mehta and S. Kapadia, "Experiences of childlessnes in an Indian context: A gender perspective," *Indian Journal of Gender Studies* 15(3) (2008): 437–460.
285. E. A. Sternke and K. Abrahamson, "Perceptions of women with infertility on stigma and disability," *Sexuality and Disability* 33(1) (2015): 3–17.
286. Sternke and Abrahamson.
287. Sternke and Abrahamson.
288. Sternke and Abrahamson.
289. B. Garner, "Mundane mommies and doting daddies: Gendered parenting and family museum visits," *Qualitative Sociology* 38(3) (2015): 327–348.
290. Gentile.
291. Garner.
292 Brooke Bass, "Preparing for parenthood?: Gender, aspirations, and the reproduction of labor market inequality," *Gender & Society* 29.3 (2015): 362–85.

293. Gentile.
294. Leire Gartzia and Janell Fetterolf, "What division of labor do university students expect in their future lives? Divergences and communalities of female and male students," *Sex Roles* 74.3–4 (2016): 121–35.
295. Fox.
296. Garner.
297. Fox.
298. Behrman.
299. Lauren Jade Martin, "Pushing for the perfect time: Social and biological fertility," *Women's Studies International Forum* 62 (2017): 91–8.
300. Belinda Diaz et al., "Transition to parenthood: The role of social interaction and endogenous networks," *Demography* 48.2 (2011): 559–79.
301. Gentile.
302. W. Chen and R. Landau, "First childbirth and motherhood at post natural fertile age: A persistent and intergenerational experience of personal and social anomaly?," *Social Work in Health Care* 54 (2015): 16–32.
303. Soderberg et al.
304. Martin.
305. Thompson and Lee.
306. C. Eriksson et al., "Reflections on fertility and postponed parenthood-interviews with highly educated women and men without children in Sweden," *Upsala Journal of Medical Sciences* 118 (2013): 122–129.
307. Martin.
308. Soderberg et al.
309. K. Benzies et al., "Factors influencing women's decisions about timing of motherhood. *The Association of Women's Health, Obstetric and Neonatal Nurses,* 35(5) (2006): 625–633.
310. Eriksson et al.
311. Chen and Landau.
312. Gentile.
313. Gentile.
314. Gentile.
315. "Celebrity post-baby bodies: Hottest before-and-after pictures," *US Weekly,* March 19, 2014, https://www.usmagazine.com/celebrity-body/pictures/hottest-celeb-post-baby-bods-20122112/36784/.
316. Jennipher Walters, "Fit moms we love: Jennifer Garner, January Jones and more!," *Shape Magazine,* https://www.shape.com/celebrities/fit-moms-we-love-jennifer-garner-january-jones-and-more.
317. Lynn O'Brien Hallstein, "Bikini-Ready Moms: Celebrity Profiles, Motherhood, and the Body," *Albany, NY: SUNY Press,* 2015.
318. Gentile.
319. Hallstein.
320. J. Maher and L. Saugeres, "To be or not to be a mother?: Women negotiating cultural representations of mothering," *Journal of Sociology,* 43(1) (2007): 5–21.
321. Sebin Song, "We Need to Talk about Kevin (2011) Trailer [Video file]," 2016, https://www.youtube.com/watch?v=ZLRgAe2jLaw.
322. Jacob Dunbar, "We Need to Talk about Kevin (2011) Trailer [Video file]," 2014, https://www.youtube.com/watch?v=ZLRgAe2jLaw.

323. S. Buerger, "The beak that grips: Maternal indifference, ambivalence and the abject in the Babadook," *Studies in Australasian Cinema, 11*(1) (2017): 33–44.

324. R. Valdrè, "We Need to Talk about Kevin": An unusual, unconventional film: Some reflections on "bad boys," between transgenerational projections and socio-cultural influences," *The International Journal of Psychoanalysis, 95*(1) (2014): 149–159.

325. Buerger.

326. S. Kornhaber, "Leaving *Neverland* Asks: What About the Parents?," *The Atlantic,* 2019, https://www.theatlantic.com/entertainment/archive/2019/03/leaving-neverland-documentary-what-parents-knew/584035/.

327. R. Riley, "Parents' Role in the Michael Jackson Trial," *NPR,* 2005, https://www.npr.org/templates/story/story.php?storyId=4628612.

328. Rosario Ceballo, Erin T. Graham, Jamie Hart, "Silent and Infertile: An Intersectional Analysis of the Experiences of Socioeconomically Diverse African American Women With Infertility," *Psychology of Women with Quarterly* 39(4) (2015): 497–511.

329. Season 8, Episode 15.

330. Season 7, Episode 16.

331. Season 8, Episode 15.

332. Season 8, Episode 1.

333. Jessica Samakow, "Olivia Pope's abortion got 1 minute of airtime—and that's all it needed," *Huffington Post,* November 20, 2015, http://www.huffingtonpost.ca/entry/olivia-popes-abortion-got-1-minute-of-airtime-and-thats-all-it-eeded_us_564e97c6e4b0879a5b0a6cc0.

334. Scott Skinner-Thompson et al., "Marriage, abortion, and coming out," *Columbia Law Review* 116 (2016): 126–51.

335. Emma Gray, "ABC wanted to cut *Scandal's* iconic abortion scene," *Huffington Post,* April 12, 2017, http://www.huffingtonpost.ca/entry/scandal-iconic-abortion-scene-abc_us_58ee37dee4b0c89f91233e44.

336. Season 7, episodes 4, 18, and 20.

337. Season 9, episode 7.

338. Mary Pols, "The Odd Life of Timothy Green: A fairy tale for the infertile," *Time,* 2012, http://entertainment.time.com/2012/08/14/the-odd-life-of-timothy-green-a-fairy-tale-for-the-infertile/.

339. Season 6, Episode 19.

340. "Internet usage frequency in Canada as of January 2017," Statista, 2018, https://www.statista.com/statistics/686835/canada-internet-usage-frequency/.

341. M. Berthelon and D.I. Kruger, "Does adolescent motherhood affect education and labor market outcomes of mothers? A study on young adult women in Chile during 1990–2013," *International Journal of Public Health 62* (2017): 293–303.

342. S.J. Gibb et al., "Early motherhood and long-term economic outcomes: Findings from a 30-year longitudinal study," *Journal of Research on Adolescence* 25(1) (2015):163–172.

343. J. Looze, "Young women's job mobility: The influence of motherhood status and education," *Journal of Marriage and Family* 76(4) (2014): 693–709.

344. Gibb et al.

345. A.R. Miller, "The effects of motherhood timing on career path." *J Popul Econ* 24 (2011): 1071–1100.

346. A. Lewin et al., "Developmental differences in parenting behavior: Comparing adolescent, emerging adult, and adult mothers," *Merrill-Palmer Quarterly* 59(1) (2013): 23–49.

347. Looze.

348. S. Frühwirth-Schnatter et al., *When is the best time to give birth?* (IZA Discussion Papers, 2014).

349. Frühwirth-Schnatter et al.

350. T. Putz and H. Engelhardt, "The effects of the first birth timing on women's wages: A longitudinal analysis based on the German Socio-Economic Panel," *Journal of Family Research* 26 (2014): 302–330.

351. J. Adda et al., "The career costs of children," (Center for Economic Studies & Ifo Institute, Working Paper no. 6158, 2016).

352. Bratti and Cavalli.

353. Adda et al.

354. Frühwirth-Schnatter et al.

355. T. Putz and H. Engelhardt, "The effects of the first birth timing on women's wages: A longitudinal analysis based on the German Socio-Economic Panel," *Journal of Family Research* 26 (2014): 302–330.

356. S. Frühwirth-Schnatter et al., *When is the best time to give birth?* (IZA Discussion Papers, 2014).

357. J. Looze, "Young women's job mobility: The influence of motherhood status and education," *Journal of Marriage and Family* 76(4) (2014): 693–709.

358. A.R. Miller, "The effects of motherhood timing on career path," *J Popul Econ* 24 (2011): 1071–1100.

359. Bratti and Cavalli.

360. Frühwirth-Schnatter.

361. Bratti and Cavalli.

362. L.M. Brown, "The relationship between motherhood and professional advancement," *Employee Relations 32*(5) (2010): 470–494.

363. J. Adda et al., "The career costs of children" (Center for Economic Studies & Ifo Institute, Working Paper no. 6158, 2016).

364. Adda et al.

365. Mikko Myrskylä and Rachel Margolis, "Happiness: Before and After the Kids," *Demography* 51(5) (2014): 1843–1866.

366. Anna Baranowska-Rataj et al., "Does Lone Motherhood Decrease Women's Happiness? Evidence from Qualitative and Quantitative Research," *Journal of Happiness Studies* 15(6) (2014): 1457–1477.

367. Nicholas H. Wolfinger, "Want to Avoid Divorce? Wait to Get Married, But Not Too Long," *Family Studies* (2015).

368. Hayford, Guzzo, and Smock.

369. OfficeTeam, "Mom To Employer: "Do You Mind If I Sit In On My Son's Interview?"," *Robert Half*, 2016, http://rh-us.mediaroom.com/2016-08-16-Mom-To-Employer-Do-You-Mind-If-I-Sit-In-On-My-Sons-Interview.

370. A. Goisis, "How are children of older mothers doing? Evidence from the United Kingdom," *Biodemography and Social Biology* 61(3) (2015): 231–251.

371. J. Fagan and Y. Lee, "Explaining the association between adolescent parenting and preschooler's school readiness: A risk perspective," *Journal of Community Psychology* 41(6) (2013): 692–708.

372. A. Lewin, "Developmental differences in parenting behavior: Comparing adolescent, emerging adult, and adult mothers," *Merrill- Palmer Quarterly* 59(1) (2013): 23–49.

373. M. Vuk, "Parenting styles and gang membership: Mediating factors," *Deviant Behavior* 38(4) (2017): 406–425.

374. Vuk.

375. Vuk.

376. L. Dillner, "What's the best age to become a mother?," *The Guardian*, March 27, 2017, https://www.theguardian.com/lifeandstyle/2017/mar/27/whats-the-best-age-to-become-a-mother.

377 Lewin et al.

378 E.V. Vugt et al., "Why is young maternal age at first childbirth a risk factor for persistent delinquency in their male offspring? Examining the role of family and parenting factors," *Criminal Behavior and Mental Health* 26 (2016): 322–335.

379. M.A. Milkie, "Does the amount of time mothers spend with children or adolescents matter?," *Journal of Marriage and Family,* 77 (2015): 355–372.

380. Vuk.

381. E. Wildsmith et al., "Teenage childbearing among youth born to teenage mothers," *Youth & Society,* 44(2) (2012): 258–283.

382. Vuk.

383. Vugt et al.

384. Y.F. Paat, "Influences of mothering and neighborhood on children's behavioral outcomes," *Children, Youth and Environment,* 20(1) (2010): 91–122.

385. S. Mollborn and J.A. Dennis, "Explaining the early development and health of teen mothers' children," *Sociological Forum,* 27(4) (2012): 1010–1036.

386. Vuk.

387. Milkie et al.

388. Wildsmith et al.

389. P.L.H. Mok et al., "Younger or older parental age and risk of suicidality, premature death, psychiatric illness, and criminality in offspring," *Journal of Affective Disorders,* 208(2016): 130–138.

390. D. Hawkes and H. Joshi, "Age at motherhood and child development: Evidence from the UK millennium cohort," *National Institute Economic Review,* 222 (2012): R52–R66.

391. Goisis.

392. Goisis.

393. Y. Rafferty et al., "Adolescent motherhood and developmental outcomes of children in Early Head Start: The influence of maternal parenting behaviors, well-being, and risk factors within the family setting," *American Journal of Orthopsychiatry,* 81(2) (2011): 228–245.

394. J. Morinis et al., "Effect of teenage motherhood on cognitive outcomes in children: a population-based cohort study," *Arch Dis Child,* 98 (2013): 959–964.

395. Fagan and Lee.

396. R. Chudal et al., "Parental age and the risk of Attention-Deficit/Hyperactivity Disorder: A nationwide, population-based cohort study," *Journal of the American Academy of Child and Adolescent Psychiatry,* 54(6) (2015): 487–495.

397. Gibb et al.

398. Mollborn and Dennis.

399. J.M. Augustine et al., "Maternal education and the link between birth timing and children's school readiness," *Social Science Quarterly*, 96(4) (2015): 970–984.

400. M. Sonobe et al., "Influence of older primiparity on childbirth, parenting stress, and mother-child interaction," *Japan Journal of Nursing Science*, 3 (2016): 229–239.

401. Mok et al.

402. Mollborn and Dennis.

403. Fagan and Lee.

404. D. Carslake et al., "Associations of parental age with health and social factors in adult offspring. Methodological pitfalls and possibilities," *Scientific Reports*, 7 (2017): 1–16.

405. Hawkes and Joshi.

406. Lewin et al.

407. D.M. Seay et al., "A prospective study of adolescent mothers' social competence, children's effortful control and compliance and children's subsequent developmental outcomes," *Social Development*, 26 (2017): 709–723.

408. Morinis et al.

409. E. Chico et al., "Executive function and mothering: Challenges faced by teenage mothers," *Developmental Psychobiology*, 56 (2014): 1027–1035.

410. Lewin et al.

411. Lewin et al.

412. Chico et al.

413. Milkie et al.

414. Chudal et al.

415. Fagan and Lee.

416. K. Barclay and M. Myrskyla, "Maternal age and offspring health and health behaviours in late adolescence in Sweden," *SSM–Population Health*, 2 (2016): 68–76.

417. M. Baker and K. Milligan, "Maternity leave and children's cognitive and behavioral development," *Journal of Population Economics, 28* (2015): 373–391.

418. Barclay and Myrskyla, *Maternal age and offspring health and health behaviours in late adolescence in Sweden.*

419. Milkie, Nomaguchi, and Denny.

420. Barclay and Myrskyla, *Maternal age and offspring health and health behaviours in late adolescence in Sweden.*

421. Goisis.

422. Goisis.

423. Carslake et al.

424. Goisis.

425. Carslake et al.

426. Myrskylä and Margolis.

427. Chudal et al.

428. G.M. Muraca et K.S. Joseph, "The association between maternal age and depression," *Journal of Obstetrics and Gynaecology Canada*, 36(9) (2014): 803–810.

429. M. Myrskyla, K. Barclay, and A. Goisis, "Advantages of later motherhood," *Der Gynäkologe*, 50 (2017): 767–772.

430. Goisis.

431. Carslake et al.

432. F.C. Billari et al., "Social age deadlines for the childbearing of women and men," *Human Reproduction, 26(3)* (2010): 616–622.
433. Muraca and Joseph.
434. M. Guedes and M.C. Canavarro, "Perceptions of influencing factors and satisfaction with the timing of first childbirth among women of advanced age and their partners," *Journal of Family Issues,* 37(13) (2016): 1797–1816.
435. Billari et al.

Bibliography

1 in 3. The 1 in 3 Campaign—These are OUR Stories. Retrieved from: http://www.1in3campaign.org/about.

Abortion Rights Network. Abortion Services Now Available in the Province of Prince Edward Island. (2017). http://www.abortionrightspei.com.

Adamczyk, A. (2008). The effects of religious contextual norms, structural constraints, and personal religiosity on abortion decisions. *Social Science Research* 37(2): 657–672.

Adda, J., et al. (2016). The career costs of children. Center for Economic Studies & Ifo Institute, Working Paper no. 6158.

Adsera, A. 2004. "Changing fertility rates in developed countries. The impact of labor market institutions." *Journal of Population Economics* 17:17–43.

Adsera, A. 2011. "Where Are the Babies? Labor Market Conditions and Fertility in Europe." *European Journal of Population* 27:1–32.

Allsworth, Jenifer E., et al. (2018) "Differences in contraceptive discontinuation among black and white women: Evidence from the Contraceptive CHOICE project." *Journal of Women's Health* 27(5): 599–606.

Ames, Christina M., and Wendy V. Norman (2012). Preventing repeat abortion in Canada: Is the immediate insertion of intrauterine devices postabortion a cost-effective option associated with fewer repeat abortions? *Contraception* 85: 51–55.

Amialchuk, A. (2013). The Effect Of Husband's Job Displacement On The Timing And Spacing Of Births In The United States, *Contemporary Economic Policy* 31(1): 73–93.

Ang, X. L. (2015). The effects of cash transfer fertility incentives and parental leave benefits on fertility and labor supply: Evidence from two natural experiments. *Journal of Family and Economic Issues*, 36(2), 263–288.

Apatow, J., Robertson, S., Townsend (Producers) & Apatow, J. (Director). (2007). *Knocked Up* [Motion picture]. United States: Universal Pictures.

Arnett, Jeffrey Jensen. 2007. "Emerging Adulthood: What Is It, and What Is It Good For?" *Child Development Perspectives* 1(2): 68–73.

Ashburn-Nardo, L. (2017). Parenthood as a moral imperative? Moral outrage and the stigmatization of voluntarily childfree women and men. *Sex Roles: A Journal of Research* 76(5–6): 393–401.

Askelson, N. M., et al. (2012). Mother–daughter communication about sex: The influence of authoritative parenting style. *Health Communication* 27(5): 439–448.

Augustine, J.M., et al. (2015). Maternal education and the link between birth timing and children's school readiness. *Social Science Quarterly*, 96(4): 970–984.

Baker, M., & Milligan, K. (2015). Maternity leave and children's cognitive and behavioral development. *Journal of Population Economics*, 28: 373–391.

Barclay, K., and Myrskylä, M. (2016). Maternal age and offspring health and health behaviours in late adolescence in Sweden. *SSM–Population Health*, 2: 68–76.

Barnes, J.C., and Morris, R.G. (2012). Young mothers, delinquent children: Assessing mediating factors among American youth. *Youth Violence and Juvenile Justice*, 10(2): 172–189.

Bartz, Deborah, and James A Greenberg (2008). Sterilization in the United States. *Reviews in Obstetrics and Gynecology* 1(1): 23–32.

Bass, Brooke. Preparing for parenthood?: Gender, aspirations, and the reproduction of labor market inequality. *Gender & Society* 29.3 (2015): 362–85.

Bassett, L. (2017). Donald Trump taps anti-contraceptive activist to oversee family planning program. *The Huffington Post*. http://www.huffingtonpost.com/entry/teresa-manning-contraception-hhs_us_5907582ae4b05c397680d921.

Baumrind, Dianna (1966). Effects of authoritative parental control on child behavior. *Child Development* 37(4): 887–907.

Bays, A. (2017). Perceptions, emotions, and behaviors toward women based on parental status. *Sex Roles*, 76: 138–155.

Beaujot, R., Du, C. J., & Ravanera, Z. (2013). Family policies in Quebec and the rest of Canada: Implications for fertility, child-care, women's paid work, and child development indicators. *Canadian Public Policy*, 39(2), 221–240.

Behrman, J.A. (2015). Does schooling affect women's desired fertility? Evidence from Malawi, Uganda, and Ethiopia. *Demography*, 52: 787–809.

Benard, S., & Correll, S. (2010). Normative discrimination and the motherhood penalty. *Gender & Society*, 24(5), 616–646.

Benson, Janel E. and Glen H. Elder Jr. "Young Adult Identities and Their Pathways: A Developmental and Life Course Model." *American Psychological Association* 47.6 (2011): 1646–1657.

Benson, Janel E., Glen H. Elder Jr. and Monica K. Johnson. "The Implications of Adult Identity for Educational and Work Attainment in Young Adulthood." *American Psychological Association* 48.6 (2011): 1752–1758.

Benzies, K., et al. (2006). Factors influencing women's decisions about timing of motherhood. *The Association of Women's Health, Obstetric and Neonatal Nurses*, 35(5): 625–633.

Bergmann, J. N., & Stockman, J. K. (2015). How does intimate partner violence affect condom and oral contraceptive use in the United States? *Contraception* 91(6): 438–455.

Bernardi, Fabrizio and Juan-Ignacio Martinez-Pastor. 2010. "Female Education and Marriage Dissolution: Is it a Selection Effect?" *European Sociological Review* 27(6): 693–707.

Berrington, Ann. (2004). Perpetual postponers? Women's, men's and couple's fertility intentions and subsequent fertility behaviour. *Population Trends*, 117, 9–19.

Bersamin, M.E., et al. (2008). Parenting practices and adolescent sexual behavior: A longitudinal study. *Journal of Marriage and Family* 70(1): 97–112.

Berthelon, M. & Kruger, D.I. (2017). *International Journal of Public Health*, 62: 293–303.

Berthelon, M., & Kruger, D.I. (2017). Does adolescent motherhood affect education and labor market outcomes of mothers? A study on young adult women in Chile during 1990-2013. *Int J Public Health*, 62: 293–303.

Billari, F.C., et al. (2010). Social age deadlines for the childbearing of women and men. *Human Reproduction, 26(3):* 616–622.

Black, Amanda, et al. (2015). "Chapter 1: Contraception in Canada." *Journal of Obstetrics and Gynaecology Canada* 37(10): S5–S12.

Black, Amanda, et al. "Chapter 1: Contraception in Canada." *Journal of Obstetrics and Gynaecology Canada* 37.10 (2015): S5–S12.

Bleakley, A., et al. (2010). Predicting preferences for types of sex education in US schools. *Sex Res Soc Policy* 7: 50–57.

Bosick, S. J. (2015). Crime and the transition to adulthood. *Crime & Delinquency, 61(7),* 950–972. doi:10.1177/0011128712461598.

Bosick, Stacey Jean. "Crime and the Transition to Adulthood: A Person-Centered Analysis of At-Risk Boys Coming of Age in 1940s Boston, 1970s London, and 1990s Pittsburgh." Diss. Harvard University, 2009.

Brand, Jennie E. and Dwight Davis. 2011. "The Impact of College Education on Fertility: Evidence for Heterogeneous Effects" *Demography* 48:863–887.

Bratti, Massimiliano and Laura Cavalli. 2014. "Delayed First Birth and New Mothers' Labor Market Outcomes: Evidence from Biological Fertility Shocks." *European Journal of Population* 30(1):35–63.

Brenning, K., Soenens, B., & Vansteenkiste, M. (2015). What's your motivation to be pregnant? Relations between motives for parenthood and women's prenatal functioning. *Journal of Family Psychology*, 29(5): 755–765.

Brentwood. (2017, October 2). *Daily Mail*. Retrieved from: http://www.dailymail.co.uk/tv-showbiz/article-4939768/Reese-Witherspoon-picks-son-karate-lessons.html.

Brinton, M. C., & Lee, D. (2016). Gender-Role ideology, labor market institutions, and Post-industrial fertility. *Population and Development Review, 42*(3), 405-433. doi:10.1111/padr.161

Brodsky, A. (2017). "Rape-adjacent": Imagining legal responses to nonconsensual condom removal. *Columbia Journal of Gender and Law* 32(2):183–210.

Brown, L. M. (2010). The relationship between motherhood and professional advancement. *Employee Relations, 32*(5), 470–494.

Brown, S. (2015). "They think it's all up to the girls": Gender, risk and responsibility for contraception. *Culture, Health & Sexuality,* 17(3): 312–325.

Brown, S. L., Manning, W. D., & Payne, K. K. (2017). Relationship quality among co-habiting versus married couples. *Journal of Family Issues, 38*(12), 1730-1753. 10.1177/0192513X15622236

Bruckner, Hannah and Karl Ulrich Mayer. "De-Standardization of the Life Course: What It Might Mean? And if It Means Anything, Whether it Actually Took Place?" *Advances in Life Course Research* 9 (2005): 27–53.

Buerger, S. (2017). The beak that grips: Maternal indifference, ambivalence and the abject in the Babadook. *Studies in Australasian Cinema, 11*(1), 33–44.

Burns, T. R., & Roszkowska, E. (2016). Rational Choice Theory: Toward a psychological, social, and material contextualization of human choice behavior. *Theoretical Economics Letters,* 6(2), 195–207.

Canadian Mental Health Association, British Columbia. (2017). Postpartum depression. Retrieved from: https://www.cmha.bc.ca/documents/postpartum-depression-3/.

Canadian Mental Health Association. (2017). Postpartum depression. Retrieved from: http://www.cmha.ca/mental_health/postpartum-depression/#.WadgcjOZNE4.

Carslake, D., et al. (2017). Associations of parental age with health and social factors in adult offspring. Methodological pitfalls and possibilities. *Scientific Reports,* 7: 1–16.

CBC (2013). Postpartum depression more common in urban areas. Retrieved from: http://www.cbc.ca/news/health/postpartum-depression-more-common-in-urban-areas-1.1409996.

CBC News. (January 19, 2011). Death penalty not on agenda. https://www.cbc.ca/news/politics/death-penalty-not-on-agenda-pm-1.1029918.

CBC News. (October 1, 2015). "Ontario sex-ed protest 'unlike anything I've ever experienced,' principal says." Retrieved from: http://www.cbc.ca/news/canada/toronto/ontario-sex-ed-protest-1.3251799.

Celebrity post-baby bodies: Hottest before-and-after pictures." (2014, March 19). *Us Weekly.* Retrieved from: https://www.usmagazine.com/celebrity-body/pictures/hottest-celeb-post-baby-bods-20122112/36784/.

Centers for Disease Control and Prevention. "Contraception." (2017). Retrieved from: https://www.cdc.gov/reproductivehealth/contraception/.

Ceyton, K. (Producer), & Kent, J. (Director). (2014). *The Babadook* [Motion picture]. Australia: Entertainment One.

Chapter 3: Emergency Contraception. *Journal of Obstetrics and Gynaecology Canada* 37(10): S20–S28.

Chavez, Paul. (2014, October 3). Super soccer mom! Denise Richards displays her impressive pitching skills as she fields an errant ball during daughter Lola's game. *Mail Online.* Retrieved from: http://www.dailymail.co.uk/tvshowbiz/article-2779064/Denise-Richards-displays-impressive-pitching-skills-fields-errant-ball-daughter-Lola-s-game.html.

Chen, W., & Landau, R. (2015). First childbirth and motherhood at post natural fertile age: A persistent and intergenerational experience of personal and social anomaly? *Social Work in Health Care,* 54:16–32.

Chico, E., et al. (2014). Executive function and mothering: Challenges faced by teenage mothers. *Developmental Psychobiology, 56:* 1027–1035.

Chudal, R., et al. (2015). Parental age and the risk of Attention-Deficit/Hyperactivity Disorder: A nationwide, population-based cohort study. *Journal of the American Academy of Child and Adolescent Psychiatry,* 54(6): 487–495.

Clack, A., & Lledo-Weber, P. (2012). Ensuring that women have access to safe abortion is "pro-life." *BMJ 345*: e4391.

Cleland, J., et al. (2014). Unmet need for contraception: Issues and challenges. *Studies in Family Planning* 45(2): 105–122.

Cohen, B. A. 1993. "Using union formation behavior to explain the transition to parenthood." Ph.D., The University of Michigan.

Connor, D. J. (2006). Michael's story: "I get into so much trouble just by walking": Narrative knowing and life at the intersections of learning disability, race, and class. *Equity & Excellence in Education, 39*(2), 154–165.

Costa, P. A., Pereira, H., & Leal, I. (2015). "The contact hypothesis" and attitudes toward same-sex parenting. *Sexuality Research & Social Policy, 12*(2), 125–136.

Davies, C. (2016, October 5). Poland's abortion ban proposal near collapse after mass protests. *The Guardian.*

Day, Jennifer C. 1994. "Age at first birth and the pacing of subsequent births: A cohort Analysis." Ph.D., The American University.

de Laat, J., & Sevilla-Sanz, A. (2011). The Fertility and Women's Labor Force Participation puzzle in OECD Countries: The Role of Men's Home Production. Feminist Economics, 17(2), 87-119. doi:10.1080/13545701.2011.573484.

De Vito, E. N. Does social stigma and personal view influence post-abortion distress? 1-105. (Order No. AAI3447720).

De Wit, Margaret L. (1993). "Educational Attainment and Timing of Childbearing among Recent Cohorts of Canadian Women." Ph.D., The University of Western Ontario.

DeCicca, Philip, and Harry Krashinsky. (2015). *Does Education Reduce Teen Fertility? Evidence from Compulsory Schooling Laws.* The National Bureau of Economic Research. Working Paper No. 21594.

Dennis, A., & Grossman, D. (2012). Barriers to contraception and interest in over-the-counter access among low-income women: A qualitative study. *Perspectives on Sexual and Reproductive Health* 44(2): 84–91.

Diaz, Belinda, et al. Transition to parenthood: The role of social interaction and endogenous networks. Demography 48.2 (2011): 559–79.

Dickerson, Bette, et al. (2012). Single mothering in poverty: Black feminist considerations, in Marcia Texler Segal et al. (eds.) *Social Production and Reproduction at the Interface of Public and Private Spheres (Advances in Gender Research, Volume 16)* (pp. 91–111). Emerald Group Publishing Limited.

Dillner, L. (2017, March 27). What's the best age to become a mother? *The Guardian.* Retrieved from: https://www.theguardian.com/lifeandstyle/2017/mar/27/whats-the-best-age-to-become-a-mother.

Dutton, I. (2013). The mother who says having these two children is the biggest regret of her life. *The Daily Mail.* Retrieved from: http://www.dailymail.co.uk/femail/article-2303588/The-mother-says-having-children-biggest-regret-life.html.

Dykstra, Pearl, and Gunhild Hagestad (2007). Roads less taken. *Journal of Family Issues* 28.10: 1275–310.

education-to-protest-at-queens-park/.

Elliott, D. B., Krivackas, K., Brault, M. W., & Kreider, R. M. (2012, May). *Historical marriage trends from 1890: A focus on race differences.* Paper presented at the 2012 annual meeting of the Population Association of America, San Francisco.

Ellis, Renee Richardson. 2010. "Interrelated Decisions? Timing of Transitions Out of Cohabitation in Relation to Other Life Course Events." Ph.D., University of California, Irvine.

Eriksson, C., et al. (2013). Reflections on fertility and postponed parenthood-interviews with highly educated women and men without children in Sweden. *Upsala Journal of Medical Sciences,* 118: 122–129.

Eriksson, Carola, Margareta Larsson, Agneta Skoog Svanberg, and Tanja Tydén. "Reflections on fertility and postponed parenthood—interviews with highly educated women and men without children in Sweden." *Upsala Journal of Medical Sciences* 118(2): 122-129.

Fagan, J., & Lee, Y. 2013. Explaining the association between adolescent parenting and preschooler's school readiness: A risk perspective. *Journal of Community Psychology*, 41(6): 692–708.

Farand, C. (2017). Man who removed condom during sex in trend known as 'stealthing' no longer found guilty of rape. *The Independent*. http://www.independent.co.uk/news/world/europe/man-remove-condom-sex-stealthing-no-conviction-rape-consent-switzerland-lausanne-a7729656.html.

Farr, R. H., et al. (2016). Microaggressions, feelings of difference, and resilience among adopted children with sexual minority parents. *Journal of Youth and Adolescence*, 45(1), 85–104.

Farrell, Justin. 2011. "The Young and the Restless? The Liberalization of Young Evangelicals." *Journal for the Scientific Study of Religion* 50(3): 517–32.

Ferre, Z., et al. (2013). The impact of teenage childbearing on educational outcomes. *The Journal of Developing Areas*, 47(2):159–174.

Ferro, M. A., and Boyle, M. H. (2015). The impact of chronic physical illness, maternal depressive symptoms, family functioning, and self-esteem on symptoms of anxiety and depression in children. *Journal of Abnormal Child Psychology*, 43: 177–187.

Ferro, M. A., et al. (2015). Association between trajectories of maternal depression and subsequent psychological functioning in youth with and without chronic physical illness. *Health Psychology*, 34(8): 820–828.

Fingerman, K. L., Kim, K., Davis, E. M., Furstenberg, F. F., Birditt, K. S., & Zarit, S. H. (2015). "I'll give you the world": Socioeconomic differences in parental support of adult children. *Journal of Marriage and Family*, 77(4), 844-865. doi:10.1111/jomf.12204

Fitch, J., et al. (2002). Condom effectiveness." *Sexually Transmitted Diseases* 29(12): 811–17.

Fletcher, J.M. (2012). The effects of teenage childbearing on the short- and long-term health behaviors of mothers. *J Popul Econ*, 25: 201–218.

Fox, B. (2001). The formative years: How parenthood creates gender. *The Canadian Review of Sociology and Anthropology*, 38(4), 373–390.

Fox, J. (Producer), & Ramsay, L. (Director). (2011). *We Need to Talk about Kevin* [Motion picture]. United Kingdom & United States: Oscilloscope Laboratories.

France, E. F., et al. (2012). Imagined futures: How experiential knowledge of disability affects parents' decision making about fetal abnormality. *Health Expectations* 15(2): 139–156.

Frejka, Tomas and Sobotka, Tomas. 2008. "Overview Chapter 1: Fertility in Europe: Diverse, delayed and below replacement." *Demographic Research*, 19(3):15–45.

Frost, J. J., et al. (2012). Young adults' contraceptive knowledge, norms and attitudes: Associations with risk of unintended pregnancy. *Perspectives on Sexual and Reproductive Health*, 44(2): 107–116.

Frühwirth-Schnatter, S., et al. (2014). When is the best time to give birth? IZA Discussion Papers.

Garner, B. (2015). Mundane mommies and doting daddies: Gendered parenting and family museum visits. *Qualitative Sociology*, 38(3), 327–348.

Gartzia, Leire, and Janell Fetterolf. What division of labor do university students expect in their future lives? Divergences and communalities of female and male students. *Sex Roles* 74.3–4 (2016): 121–35.

Gaudet, S., Cooke, M., & Jacob, J. (2011). Working after childbirth: A lifecourse transition analysis of Canadian women from the 1970s to the 2000s. *Canadian Review of Sociology/ Revue canadienne de sociologie*, 48(2), 153–180.

Gauthier, Anne H. 2002. "Family Policies in Industrialized Countries: Is There Convergence?" *Population* 57(3):447–474.

Gauthier, Anne H. 2007. "The impact of family policies on fertility in industrialized countries: A review of the literature." *Population Research and Policy Review* 26: 323–346.

Gentile, K. (2011). Reply to commentaries: "What about the baby? The new cult of domesticity and media images of pregnancy." *Studies in Gender and Sexuality*, 12(1), 72–77.

Ghimire, Dirgha. 2015. "Wives' and Husbands' Nonfamily Experiences and First-Birth Timing." *International Journal of Sociology* 45(1): 4–23.

Gibb, S.J., et al. (2015). Early motherhood and long-term economic outcomes: Findings from a

30-year longitudinal study. *Journal of Research on Adolescence*, 25(1):163–172.

Gilleard, Chris and Paul Higgs. 2016. "Connecting Life Span Development with the Sociology of the Life Course: A New Direction." *Sociligy* 50(2): 301-315.

Gillin, C.T. and Thomas R. Klassen. "Retire Mandatory Retirement." *Policy Options* (2000): 59–62.

Goisis, A. (2015). How are children of older mothers doing? Evidence from the United Kingdom. *Biodemography and Social Biology* 61(3): 231–251.

Gordon, M., & Cui, M. (2015). Positive parenting during adolescence and career success in young adulthood. *Journal of Child and Family Studies, 24*(3), 762-771. doi:10.1007/s10826-013-9887-y

Government of Canada, Department of Justice, Electronic Communications. 2015. "Custody, Access and Child Support: Findings from The National Longitudinal Survey of Children and Youth." *Government of Canada, Department of Justice, Electronic Communications.* Retrieved February 1, 2018 (http://www.justice.gc.ca/eng/rp-pr/fl-lf/famil/anlsc-elnej/p2_01.html).

Grace, K., & Anderson, J. (2016). Reproductive coercion: A systemic review. *Trauma, Violence, and Abuse*: 1–20. doi: 10.1177/1524838016663935.

Graham, R. (2016). The Myth of Abortion Regret. *Slate*. http://www.slate.com/articles/double_x/doublex/2016/10/the_myth_of_abortion_regret.html.

Gray, Emma. (2017, April 12). ABC wanted to cut *Scandal*'s iconic abortion scene. *Huffington Post*. Retrieved from http://www.huffingtonpost.ca/entry/scandal-iconic-abortion-scene-abc_us_58ee37dee4b0c89f91233e44.

Grey's Anatomy (2005–2017). Shonda Rhimes. American Broadcasting Company.

Grossman, J.M., et al. (2014). Protective effects of middle school comprehensive sex education with family involvement. *Journal of School Health*, 84(11): 739–747.

Guedes, M., & Canavarro, M. C. (2016). Perceptions of influencing factors and satisfaction with the timing of first childbirth among women of advanced age and their partners. *Journal of Family Issues*, 37(13): 1797–1816.

Haan, Peter and Katharina Wrohlich. 2011. "Can Child Care Policy Encourage Employment and Fertility? Evidence from a Structural Model." *Labour Economics* 18: 498–512.

Halle, Claire, et al. (2008). Supporting fathers in the transition to parenthood. *Contemporary Nurse*, 31(1): 57ff.

Hallstein, Lynn O'Brien. (2015). *Bikini-Ready Moms: Celebrity Profiles, Motherhood, and the Body*. Albany, NY: SUNY Press.

Hammer, Muriel, Linda Gutwirth, and Susan L. Phillips. Parenthood and social networks. *Social Science and Medicine* 16.24 (1982): 2091–100.

Hanschmidt, F., et al. (2016). Abortion stigma: A systemic review. *Perspectives on Sexual and Reproductive Health*. 48(4): 169–177.

Hansen, Thomas. Parenthood and happiness: A review of folk theories versus empirical evidence. *Social Indicators Research* 108.1 (2012): 29–64.

Hawkes, D., and Joshi, H. (2012). Age at motherhood and child development: Evidence from the UK millennium cohort. *National Institute Economic Review*, 222: R52–R66.

Hayford, S.R., Guzzo, K.N., & Smock, P.J. (2014). The decoupling of marriage and parenthood? Trends in the timing of marital first births, 1945-2002. *Journal of Marriage and Family*, 76(3), 520-538. doi: 10.1111/jomf.12114

Hayford, Sarah R., Karen Benjamin Guzzo, and Pamela J. Smock. 2014. "The Decoupling of Marriage and Parenthood? Trends in the Timing of Marital First Births, 1945-2002." *Journal of Marriage and Family* 76(3): 520–38.

Held, L., & Rutherford, A. (2012). Can't a mother sing the blues? Postpartum depression and the construction of motherhood in late 20th-century America. *History of Psychology*, 15(2), 107–123.

Herold, S., et al. (2015). Women's private conversations about abortion: A qualitative study. *Women & Health*, 55(8): 943–959.

Heuveline, Patrick and Jeffrey M. Timberlake. 2004. "The role of cohabitation in family formation: The United States in Comparative Perspective." *Journal of Marriage and Family* 66(5): 1214-1230.

Hilgeman, Christin and Carter T Butts. 2009. "Women's employment and fertility: A welfare regime paradox." *Social Science Research* 38(1): 103-117.

Hitchens, B. K., & Payne, Y. A. (2017). "Brenda's got a baby". *Journal of Black Psychology, 43*(1), 50-76. 10.1177/0095798415619260

Hofmeister, H. (2013). Individualisation of the life course. *International Social Science Journal, 64*(213-214), 279-290. doi:10.1111/issj.12053

Hogan, Dennis P. 1980. "The Transition to Adulthood as a Career Contingency." *American Sociological Review* 45(2):261–276.

Howell, Nancy (1969). *The Search for an Abortionist.* Chicago: University of Chicago Press. http://planb.ca

Hurford, E., et al. (2013). The decision to continue a pregnancy affected by Down syndrome: Timing of decision and satisfaction with receiving a prenatal diagnosis. *Journal of Genetic Counseling, 22*(5): 587–593.

Hussey, L. S. (2010). Welfare generosity, abortion access, and abortion rates: A comparison of state policy tools. *Social Science Quarterly* 91(1): 266–283.

Iacovou, Maria and Tavares, Lara Patrício. (2011). Yearning, Learning, and Conceding: Reasons Men and Women Change Their Childbearing Intentions. *Population and Development Review,* 37(1): 89-123

Ibisomi, L., & Mudege, N.N. (2014) Childlessness in Nigeria: perceptions and acceptability. *Culture, Health & Sexuality,* 16(1): 61–75.

Inanc, H. (2015). Unemployment and the timing of parenthood: Implications of partnership status and partner's employment. *Demographic Research, 219.* doi: 10.4054/DemRes.2015.32.7

Jacob Dunbar. (2014). Re: *We Need to Talk about Kevin (2011) Trailer* [Video file]. Retrieved from https://www.youtube.com/watch?v=ZLRgAe2jLaw.

Jennings, Elyse. (2013). The Influence of Wives' and Husbands' Fertility Preferences on Progression to Higher Parity Pregnancies in Nepal. *Population Association of America.*

Jones, R., & Frohwirth, L. (2013). More than poverty: disruptive events among women having abortions in the USA. *The Journal of Family Planning and Reproductive Health Care* 39(1): 36.

Jutte, D. P., et al. (2010). The ripples of adolescent motherhood: Social, educational, and medical outcomes for children of teen and prior teen mothers. *Academic Pediatrics,* 10(5): 293–301.

Kahn, J.R., et al. (2014). The motherhood penalty at midlife: Long-term effects of children on women's careers. *Journal of Marriage and Family,* 76: 56–72.

Kalb, G., et al. (2015). Outcomes for teenage mothers in the first years after birth. *Australian Journal of Labour Economics,* 18(3): 255–279.

Kaposy, Chris (2010). Improving Abortion Access in Canada. *Health Care Analysis* 18: 17–34.

Karimi, A. (2014). Effects of the timing of births on women's earnings: Evidence from a natural experiment. Working Paper, IFAU, Institute for Evaluation of Labour Market and Education Policy, No. 2014:17.

Kemnitz, A., & Thum, M. (2015). Gender power, fertility, and family Policy1. *The Scandinavian Journal of Economics, 117*(1), 220-247. 10.1111/sjoe.12086

Kemnitz, A., & Thum, M. (2015). Gender power, fertility, and family Policy1. *The Scandinavian Journal of Economics, 117*(1), 220-247. 10.1111/sjoe.12086

Khazan, O. (2017, May 22). How people decide whether to have children. *The Atlantic.* https://www.theatlantic.com/health/archive/2017/05/how-people-   decide-whether-to-have-children/527520/.

Kiernan, Kathleen. 2004. "Unmarried Cohabitation and Parenthood in Britain and Europe." *Law & Policy* 26(1): 33-55.

Kimport, K., et al. (2012). Addressing the silence in the noise: How abortion support talklines meet some women's needs for non-political discussion of their experiences. *Women & Health* 52(1): 88–100.

Kohli, Martin. "The Institutionalization of the Life Course: Looking Back to Look Ahead." *Research in Human Development* 4.3 (2007): 253–271.

Kohn, J. (2014). Five-year trends in medication abortion: A view from planned parenthood. *Contraception* 89.5 (2014): 479–.

Kok, Jan. "Principles and Prospects of the Life Course Paradigm." *Annales de Demographie Historique* 1 (2007): 203–230.

Kornhaber, S. (2019). *The Atlantic. Leaving Neverland* Asks: What About the Parents? Retrieved from https://www.theatlantic.com/entertainment/archive/2019/03/leaving-neverland-documentary-what-parents-knew/584035/.

Kulu, Hill and Paul J. Boyle. 2010. "Premarital cohabitation and divorce: Support for "Trial Marriage" Theory?" *Demographic Research* 23(31): 879-904.

Lamidi, E. & Manning, W. D. (2016). FP-16-17 Marriage and Cohabitation Experiences Among Young Adults. https://www.bgsu.edu/ncfmr/resources/data/family-profiles/lamidi-manning-marriage-cohabitation-young-adults-fp-16-17.html.

Lamont, E. (2014). Negotiating courtship: Reconciling egalitarian ideals with traditional gender norms. *Gender & Society, 28*(2), 189-211. 10.1177/0891243213503899

Langdridge, D., Sheeran, P., & Connolly, K. (2005). Understanding the reasons for parenthood. *Journal of Reproductive and Infant Psychology,* 23(2): 121–133.

Lanre-Babalola, F. (2015). Dynamics of knowledge, use and preference of birth control methods among women of reproductive age in urban areas. *International Journal of Innovation and Applied Studies* 13(1): 137–45.

Laplante, Benoit. The well-being of families in Canada's future. *Canadian Studies in Population,* 1.2, 24–32.

Lewin, A., et al. (2013). Developmental differences in parenting behavior: Comparing adolescent, emerging adult, and adult mothers. *Merrill- Palmer Quarterly,* 59(1): 23–49.

Lindell, Rebecca and Young, Leslie. 2012. "Meet the boomerang kids: 40% of young adults living with their parents." *Global News.* Retrieved from: http://globalnews.ca/news/288198/meet-the-boomerang-kids-40-of-young-adults-living-with-their-parents/.

Little, T., et al. (2010). Perceptions of teen pregnancy among high school students in Sweet Home, Oregon. *Health Education Journal* 69(3): 333–343.

Lobel, M. & Rosenthal, L. (2016). Stereotypes of Black American women related to sexuality and motherhood. *Psychology of Women Quarterly,* 40(3): 414–427.

Looze, J. (2014). Young women's job mobility: The influence of motherhood status and education. *Journal of Marriage and Family,* 76(4): 693–709.

Looze, Jessica. 2014. "Young Womens Job Mobility: The Influence of Motherhood Status and Education." *Journal of Marriage and Family* 76(4): 693–709.

Luci-Greulich, A., & Thévenon, O. (2013). The impact of family policies on fertility trends in developed countries. *European Journal of Population / Revue Européenne De Démographie,* 29(4), 387-416.

Lupton, D. (2000). "A love/hate relationship": The ideals and experiences of first-time mothers. *Journal of Sociology, 36*(1), 50–63.

Lupton, D. (2000). A love/hate relationship: The ideals and experiences of first-time mothers. *Journal of Sociology, 36*(1), 50–63.

Lutz, Wolfgang and Samir, KC. 2011. "Global Human Capital: Integrating Education and Population." *Science* 333(6042): 587–92.

Lyubomirsky, S., & Boehm, J.K. (2010). Human Motives, Happiness, and the Puzzle of Parenthood: Commentary on Kenrick et al. *Perspectives on Psychological Science,* 5(3): 327–334.

Macmillan, Ross. "The Structure of the Life Course: Classic Issues and Current Controversies." *Advances in Life Course Research* 9 (2005): 3–24.

Maher, J., & Saugeres, L. (2007). To be or not to be a mother?: Women negotiating cultural representations of mothering. *Journal of Sociology,* 43(1), 5–21.

Maher, J., & Saugeres, L. (2007). To be or not to be a mother?: Women negotiating cultural representations of mothering. *Journal of Sociology,* 43(1), 5–21.

Malacrida, C., & Boulton, T. (2012). Women's perceptions of childbirth "choices": Competing discourses of motherhood, sexuality, and selflessness. *Gender and Society, 26*(5), 748–772.

Martin, Lauren Jade (2017). Pushing for the perfect time: Social and biological fertility. *Women's Studies International Forum* 62: 91–8.

McKnight, Z. (2017, January 31). Don't worry, you can still get an IUD in Canada—if you have insurance. *Toronto Star.*

Mehta, B., Kapadia, S. (2008). Experiences of childlessnes in an Indian context: A gender perspective. *Indian Journal of Gender Studies, 15*(3): 437–460.

Metcalfe, A., et al. (2016). Exploring the relationship between socioeconomic factors, method of contraception and unintended pregnancy. *Reproductive Health* 13(28): 1–8.

Metcalfe, A., Vekved, M., & Tough, S. (2014). Educational attainment, perception of workplace support and its influence on timing of childbearing for canadian women: A cross-sectional study. *Maternal and Child Health Journal, 18*(7), 1675-1682. doi:10.1007/s10995-013-1409-4

Meyer, D., et al. (2016). The possible trajectory of relationship satisfaction across the longevity of a romantic partnership: Is there a golden age of parenting? *The Family Journal, 24*(4): 344 – 350.

Milan, Anne. 2016. "Insights on Canadian Society Diversity of young adults living with their parents." *Statistics Canada.* Retrieved from: http://www.statcan.gc.ca/pub/75-006-x/2016001/article/14639-eng.htm.

Milkie, M. A., et al. (2015). Does the amount of time mothers spend with children or adolescents matter? *Journal of Marriage and Family, 77*: 355–372.

Milkie, M. A., et al. (2015). Does the amount of time mothers spend with children or adolescents matter? *Journal of Marriage and Family, 77*: 355–372.

Milkie, M. A., et al. (2016). What kind of war? "Mommy wars" discourse in U.S. and Canadian news, 1989–2013. *Sociological Inquiry,* 86(1): 51–78.

Milkie, M. A., Pepin, J. R., & Denny, K. E. (2016). What kind of war? "Mommy wars" discourse in U.S. and canadian news, 1989–20131. *Sociological Inquiry,* 86(1), 51-78. 10.1111/soin.12100

Milkie, M.A., et al. (2015). Does the amount of time mothers spend with children or adolescents matter? *Journal of Marriage and Family, 77*: 355–372.

Miller, A. R. (2011). The effects of motherhood timing on career path. *Journal of Population Economics, 24*(3), 1071-1100.

Miller, A.R. (2011). The effects of motherhood timing on career path. *J Popul Econ,* 24: 1071–1100.

Millner, V., et al. (2015). Parents' beliefs regarding sex education for their children in Southern Alabama public schools. *Sex Res Soc Policy* 12: 101–109.

Mills, M., et al. (2011). Why do people postpone parenthood? Reasons and social policy incentives. *Human Reproduction Update,* 17(6): 848–860.

Mills, Melinda, Ronald R. Rindfuss, Peter McDonald, and Egbert te Velde. 2011. "Why do people postpone parenthood? Reasons and social policy incentives." *Human Reproduction Update* 17(6): 848–860.

Ministry of Health and Long-Term Care. (2017). Initial Report on Public Health: Teen Pregnancy. http://www.health.gov.on.ca/en/public/publications/pubhealth/init_report/tp.html.

Mok, P. L. H., et al. (2016). Younger or older parental age and risk of suicidality, premature death, psychiatric illness, and criminality in offspring. *Journal of Affective Disorders,* 208(2017): 130–138.

Mollborn, S., & Dennis, J.A. (2011). Investigating the life situations and development of teenage mother's children: Evidence from ECLS-B. *Popul Res Policy Rev,* 31: 31–66.

Mollborn, S., & Dennis, J.A. (2012). Explaining the early development and health of teen mothers' children. *Sociological Forum,* 27(4): 1010–1036.

Moller, K., Hwang, C.P., Wickberg, B. (2008). Couple relationship and transition to parenthood: Does workload at home matter? *Journal of Reproductive and Infant Psychology,* 26(1): 57–68.

Montgomery, K.S., et al. (2010). Women's desire for pregnancy. *The Journal of Perinatal Education*, 19(3): 53–61.

Moreira, T. (2016). De-standardising ageing? shifting regimes of age measurement. *Ageing and Society*, 36(7), 1407-1433. doi:10.1017/S0144686X15000458

Morinis, J., et al. (2013). Effect of teenage motherhood on cognitive outcomes in children: a population-based cohort study. *Arch Dis Child*, 98: 959–964.

Mossakowski, Krysia N. "Unfulfilled expectations and symptoms of depression among young adults." *Social Science and Medicine* 73 (2011): 729–736.

Motro, J. and Vanneman, R. (2015), The 1990s shift in the media portrayal of working mothers. *Social Forum*, 30: 1017–1037.

Muhammad, A., & Gagnon, A. (2010). Why should men and women marry and have children? Parenthood, marital status and self perceived stress among Canadians. *Journal of Health Psychology*, 15(3): 315–325.

Muraca, G.M., and Joseph, K.S. (2014). The association between maternal age and depression. *Journal of Obstetrics and Gynaecology Canada*, 36(9): 803–810.

Myrskyla, M., et al. (2017). Advantages of later motherhood. *Der Gynäkologe*, 50: 767–772.

Myrskylä, M., Goldstein, J. R., & Cheng, Y. A. (2013). New cohort fertility forecasts for the developed world: Rises, falls, and reversals. *Population and Development Review*, 39(1), 31-56. doi:10.1111/j.1728-4457.2013.00572.x

Nádasi, Eszter (2016). Changing the face of medicine, alternating the meaning of human. *Critical Studies in Television: The International Journal of Television Studies* 11(2): 230–43.

Neels, Karel and David De Wachter. 2010. "Postponement and recuperation of Belgian fertility: how are they related to rising female educational attainment?." *Vienna Yearbook of Population Research* 8: 77-106.

Nelson, S.K., et al. (2013). In defense of parenthood: Children are associated with more joy than misery. *Psychological Science*, 24(1):3–10.

Nichols, L. J. (2016). Motherhood and unemployment: Intersectional experiences from Canada. *Canadian Review of Social Policy* 76: 1–24.

Nico, Magda. "Individualized Housing Careers in Early Adulthood: Conditions and Constraints in a Familistic Society." *Sociological Research Online* 15.1 (2010).

Nico, Magda. 2014. "Variability in the the transitions to adulthood in Europe: a critical approach to de-standardization of the life course" *Journal of Youth Studies* 17(2): 166-182.

Norton, A. (2012). "Women overestimate effectiveness of the pill, condoms." *Toronto Star*. https://www.thestar.com/life/health_wellness/2012/04/27/women_overestimate_effectiveness_of_the_pill_condoms.html.

Nuccetelli, Susana. (2017) "Abortion for fetal defects: Two current arguments." *Medicine, Health Care and Philosophy* 20 (3): 447–450.

Ochiogu, I. N., et al. (2011). Impact of sex education on teenage pregnancy in Nigeria: Cross-sectional survey of secondary school students. *J Community Health* 36: 375–380.

OfficeTeam. (2016). Mom To Employer: "Do You Mind If I Sit In On My Son's Interview?" Retrieved from http://rh-us.mediaroom.com/2016-08-16-Mom-To-Employer-Do-You-Mind-If-I-Sit-In-On-My-Sons-Interview.

O'Hara, M. (2009, September 23). Thirty is the new mom. *Metro*. Retrieved from http://www.metronews.ca/news/2009/09/23/thirty-is-the-new-mom.html.

OHIP+. Learn About OHIP+. Retrieved from <https://www.ontario.ca/page/learn-about-ohip-plus>.

Ou, S., & Reynolds, A. (2013). Timing of first childbirth and young Women's postsecondary education in an inner-city minority cohort. *Urban Education*, 48(2), 289-313. doi:10.1177/0042085912451586

Paat, Y. F. (2010). Influences of mothering and neighborhood on children's behavioral outcomes. *Children, Youth and Environment*, 20(1): 91–122.

Panek, Paul E., Sara Staats and Amanda Hiles. "College Students' Perceptions of Job Demands, Recommended Retirement Ages, and Age of Optimal Performance in Selected Occupations." *International Journal of Aging and Human Development* 62.2 (2006): 87–115.

Patel, A. (2017). Mothers talk candidly about postpartum depression: "You're not alone." *Global News*. http://globalnews.ca/news/3417263/postpartum-depression-signs/

Paull, G. (2014). Can government intervention in childcare be justified? *Economic Affairs, 34*(1), 14-34.

Perelli-Harris, Brienna and Nora Sanchez Gassen. 2012. "How Similar Are Cohabitation and Marriage? Legal Approaches to Cohabitation across Western Europe." *Population and Development Review* 38(3): 435–467.

Philipov, Liefbroer, Klobas, *Reproductive Decision-Making in a Macro-Micro Perspective*, 2015.

Planned Parenthood. "Birth Control Implant." *Planned Parenthood*. (2017). Retrieved from: https://www.plannedparenthood.org/learn/birth-control/birth-control-implant-implanon.

Planned Parenthood. "Birth Control Methods." Planned Parenthood.org. N.p., n.d. Web.

Planned Parenthood. "IUD." *Planned Parenthood*. (2017). Retrieved from: https://www.plannedparenthood.org/learn/birth-control/iud.

Planned Parenthood. "Morning-After Pill (Emergency Contraception)." (2017). Retrieved from: https://www.plannedparenthood.org/learn/morning-after-pill-emergency-contraception

Pols, Mary. (2012). "*The Odd Life of Timothy Green*: A fairy tale for the infertile." *Time*. Retrieved from http://entertainment.time.com/2012/08/14/the-odd-life-of-timothy-green-a-fairy-tale-for-the-infertile/.

Putz, T., & Engelhardt, H. (2014). The effects of the first birth timing on women's wages: A longitudinal analysis based on the German Socio-Economic Panel. *Journal of Family Research, 26*: 302–330.

Rackin, H.M., and Brasher, M.S. (2016). Is baby a blessing? Wantedness, age at first birth, and later-life depression. *Journal of Marriage and Family*, 78(5): 1269–1284.

Rafferty, Y., et al. (2011). Adolescent motherhood and developmental outcomes of children in Early Head Start: The influence of maternal parenting behaviors, well-being, and risk factors within the family setting. *American Journal of Orthopsychiatry*, 81(2): 228–245.

Ralph, L. J., et al. (2017). Measuring decisional certainty among women seeking abortion. *Contraception* 95: 269–278.

Reddit. https://www.reddit.com/r/Parenting/comments/1wvx04/serious_do_you_regret_having_children/?sort=confidence.

Riley, R. (2005). *Parents' Role in the Michael Jackson Trial*. NPR. Retrieved from https://www.npr.org/templates/story/story.php?storyId=4628612.

Rindfuss, R., Choe, M., & Brauner-Otto, S. (2016). The emergence of two distinct fertility regimes in economically advanced countries. *Population Research and Policy Review, 35*(3), 287-304. doi:10.1007/s11113-016-9387-z

Rocca, C.H., et al. (2013). Young women's perceptions of the benefits of childbearing: Associations with contraceptive use and pregnancy. *Perspectives on Sexual and Reproductive Health*, 45(1): 23–32.

Rocca, Corinne H., et al. (2015). Decision rightness and emotional responses to abortion in the United States: A longitudinal study. *PLOS One*. Retrieved from: http://journals.plos.org/plosone/article?id=10.1371/journal.pone.0128832#sec014.

Ryan, S., et al. (2007). Adolescents' discussions about contraception or STDs with partners before first sex. *Perspectives on Sexual and Reproductive Health* 39(3): 149–157.

Samakow, Jessica. (2015, November 20). Olivia Pope's abortion got 1 minute of airtime—and that's all it needed. *Huffington Post*. Retrieved from http://www.huffingtonpost.ca/entry/olivia-popes-abortion-got-1-minute-of-airtime-and-thats-all-it-eeded_us_564e97c6e-4b0879a5b0a6cc0.

Saunders, D. (2007). I really regret it. I really regret having children. *The Globe and Mail*. https://www.theglobeandmail.com/life/parenting/mothers-day/i-really-regret-it-i-really-regret-having-children/article1200668/?page=all.

Schmitz, D. (2012). Terminating pregnancy after prenatal diagnosis–with a little help of professional ethics? *Journal of Medical Ethics* 38: 399–402.

Scott, S & Lei-Lei, J. (2015). Failures-to-launch and boomerang kids: Contemporary determinants of leaving and returning to the parental home. *Social Forces, 94*(2), 863.

Seay, D. M., et al. (2017). A prospective study of adolescent mothers' social competence, children's effortful control and compliance and children's subsequent developmental outcomes. *Social Development,* 26: 709–723.

Sebin Song. (2016). Re: *We Need to Talk about Kevin (2011) Trailer* [Video file]. Retrieved from https://www.youtube.com/watch?v=ZLRgAe2jLaw.

Shandra, C. L., et al. (2014). Planning for motherhood: Fertility attitudes, desires and intentions among women with disabilities. *Perspectives on Sexual and Reproductive Health, 46*(4), 203–210.

Shea, R., et al. (2016). "Nappy bags instead of handbags": Young motherhood and self-identity. *Journal of Sociology, 52*(4), 840–855.

Silent No More Awareness. About Us. Retrieved from: http://www.silentnomoreawareness.org/about-us/index.aspx.

Silk, Jessica, and Diana Romero (2014). The role of parents and families in teen pregnancy prevention: An analysis of programs and policies. *Journal of Family Issues* 35 (10): 1339–1362.

Skinner-Thompson, Scott, et al. (2016). Marriage, abortion, and coming out. *Columbia Law Review* 116: 126–51.

Smith, J. L., et al. (2012). Perceptions of teen motherhood in Australian adolescent females: Life-line or life derailment. *Women and Birth, 25*(4), 181–186.

Sobotka, T., Skirbekk, V., & Philipov, D. (2011). Economic recession and fertility in the developed world. *Population and Development Review, 37*(2), 267-306. doi:10.1111/j.1728-4457.2011.00411.x

Sobotka, Tomáš, and Äva Beaujouan (2017). Late motherhood in low-fertility countries: Reproductive intentions, trends and consequences. *Preventing Age Related Fertility Loss,* doi:10.1007/978-3-319-14857-1_2.

Soderberg, M., et al. (2015). Women's attitudes towards fertility and childbearing: A study based on a national sample of Swedish women validating the Attitudes to Fertility and Childbearing Scale (AFCS). *Sexual & Reproductive Healthcare,* 1–5.

Sonobe, M., et al. (2016). Influence of older primiparity on childbirth, parenting stress, and mother-child interaction. *Japan Journal of Nursing Science,* 3: 229–239.

Statista. Internet usage frequency in Canada as of January 2017. Retrieved from https://www.statista.com/statistics/686835/canada-internet-usage-frequency/.

Statistics Canada. (2015). *Communications Monitoring Report 2015: Canada's Communications System: An Overview for Citizens, Consumers, and Creators.*

Statistics Canada. (2017). *CANSIM Table 102-4505, Births and total fertility rate, by province and territory (Fertility rate).* Retrieved from https://www.statcan.gc.ca/tables-tableaux/sum-som/l01/cst01/hlth85b-eng.htm.

Sternke, E. A., & Abrahamson, K. (2015). Perceptions of women with infertility on stigma and disability. *Sexuality and Disability, 33*(1), 3–17.

Stevens, L.M. (2015). Planning parenthood: Health care providers' perspectives on pregnancy intention, readiness, and family planning. *Social Science & Medicine,* 139: 44–52.

Stewart, Mary, and Kirsten Black (2015). Choosing a combined oral contraceptive pill. *Australian Prescriber* **38(1): 6–11.**

Stone, Juliet, Ann Berrington, and Jane Falkingham. 2011. "The changing determinants of UK young adults' living arrangements." *Demographic Research* 25: 629–66.

Stranger-Hall, Kathrin F., and David W. Hall (2011). Abstinence-only education and teen pregnancy rates: Why we need comprehensive sex education in the U.S." *PLoS ONE* 6(10): e24658–e24658.

Testa, Maria Rita, Cavalli, Laura, and Rosina, Alessandro. (2014). The Effect of Couple Disagreement about Child-Timing Intentions: A Parity-Specific Approach. *Population and Development Review.*

The Canadian Press. (2016, September 21). Parents against sex education to protest at Queen's Park. *City News.* http://www.citynews.ca.

Thévenon, O., & Gauthier, A. H. (2011). Family policies in developed countries: a 'fertility-booster' with side-effects. *Community, Work & Family, 14*(2), 197-216.

Thompson, R., & Lee, C. (2011). Sooner or later? Young Australian men's perspectives on timing of parenthood. *Journal of Health Psychology,* 16(5): 807–818.

Thomson, Elizabeth. "Family Complexity in Europe." *The ANNALS of the American Academy of Political and Social Science,* 654(1): 245-58.

Thornicroft, K.W. (2016). The Uncertain State of Mandatory Retirement in Canada. *Labour and Law Journal,* 67(2), 397-414.

Thorton, Arland and Linda Young-DeMarco. 2004. "Four Decades of Trends in Attitudes Toward Family Issues in the United States: The 1960s Through the 1990s." *Journal of Marriage and Family* 63: 1009-1037.

Tomasi, P. (2017). A massive postpartum depression study has just opened in Canada. *The Huffington Post.* http://www.huffingtonpost.ca/2017/04/27/postpartum-depression-study_n_16272462.html.

Tousignant, L. (2017). 'Stealthing' is the newest dangerous sex trend. *New York Post.* Retrieved from: http://nypost.com/2017/04/24/stealthing-is-the-newest-dangerous-sex-trend/.

Trimarci, A. & Van Bevel, J. (2017). Education and the transition into fatherhood: The role of selection into union. *Demography, 54,* 119-144. doi: 10.1007/s13524-016-0533-3

Tucker, J. S., et al. (2012). Understanding pregnancy-related attitudes and behaviors: A mixed-methods study of homeless youth. *Perspectives on Sexual and Reproductive Health* 44(4): 252–261.

Valdrè, R. (2014). "We Need to Talk about Kevin": An unusual, unconventional film: Some reflections on "bad boys," between transgenerational projections and socio-cultural influences. *The International Journal of Psychoanalysis,* 95(1), 149–159.

Vincent, K., & Thomson, P. (2013). "Your age don't determine whether you're a good mum": Reframing the discourse of deviance ascribed to teenage mothers. *Social Alternatives,* 32(2), 6–12.

Voas, David. (2003). Conflicting Preferences: A Reason Fertility Tends to Be Too High or Too Low. *Population and Development Review,* 29 (4): 627–646.

Vugt, E.V., et al. (2016). Why is young maternal age at first childbirth a risk factor for persistent delinquency in their male offspring? Examining the role of family and parenting factors. *Criminal Behavior and Mental Health,* 26: 322–335.

Vuk, M. 2017. Parenting styles and gang membership: Mediating factors. *Deviant Behavior,* 38(4): 406–425.

Wakefield, J., et al. (2016). The nation and the family: The impact   of national identification and perceived importance of family values on homophobic attitudes in Lithuania and Scotland. *Sex Roles,* 75(9–10), 448–458.

Waldfogel, J. (2016). How important is parental time? It depends: Comment on Milkie, Nomaguchi, and Denny (2015). *Journal of Marriage and Family,* 78(1): 266–269.

Wall-Wieler, Elizabeth, et al. (2016). Teenage pregnancy: The impact of maternal adolescent childbearing and older sister's teenage pregnancy on a younger sister." *BMC Pregnancy and Childbirth* 16(1): 120–132.

Walters, Jennipher (n.d.). "Fit moms we love: Jennifer Garner, January Jones and more! *Shape Magazine.* Retrieved from https://www.shape.com/celebrities/fit-moms-we-love-jennifer-garner-january-jones-and-more.

Webb, R.T., et al. (2011). Teenage motherhood and risk of premature death: Long-term follow-up in the ONS Longitudinal Study. *Psychological Medicine,* 41: 1867–1877.

Weiss, Jessica. 2000. *To Have and to Hold: Marriage, the Baby Boom, and Social Change.* Chicago: University of Chicago Press.

Weitz, T. A. (2010). Rethinking the mantra that abortion should be "safe, legal, and rare." *Journal of Women's History* 22(3): 161–172.

Wiebe, E. (2013). Contraceptive practices and attitudes among immigrant and nonimmigrant women in Canada. *Canadian Family Physician* 59(10): 451–455.

Wilde, M., & Danielsen, S. (2014). Fewer and better children: Race, class, religion, and birth control reform in America. *American Journal of Sociology* 119(6): 1710–1760.

Wildsmith, E., et al. (2012). Teenage childbearing among youth born to teenage mothers. *Youth & Society*, 44(2): 258–283.

Wildsmith, E., et al. (2015). Relationship characteristics and contraceptive use among dating and cohabiting young adult couples. *Perspectives on Sexual and Reproductive Health* 47(1): 27–36.

Williams, C., et al. (2008). Intimate partner violence and women's contraceptive use. *Violence Against Women* 14(12): 1382–1396.

Worts, D., Sacker, A., McMunn, A., & McDonough, P. (2013). Individualization, opportunity and jeopardy in american women's work and family lives: A multi-state sequence analysis. *Advances in Life Course Research, 18*(4), 296-318. 10.1016/j.alcr.2013.09.003

Wulfhost, E. (2017, May 3). Teenage pregnancies rise in Guatemala as girls are deprived of basic sex education warn healthcare campaigners. *The Independent*. Retrieved from: http://www.independent.co.uk/news/world/americas/teenage-pregnancies-guatemala-girls-basic-sex-education-contraception-violence-healthcare-a7715406.html.

Wyatt, Frederick (1971). A clinical view of parenthood. *Bulletin of the Menninger Clinic* 35.3: 167.

Yen, Sophia, et al. (2015). Emergency contraception pill awareness and knowledge in uninsured adolescents: High rates of misconceptions concerning indications for use, side effects, and access. *Journal of Pediatric and Adolescent Gynecology* 28(5): 337–42.

Index